Let's Get
It On

Let's Get
It On

*15 Hot Tips and Tricks
to Spice Up Your Sex Life*

LaDawn Black

ONE WORLD
BALLANTINE BOOKS/NEW YORK

A One World Books Trade Paperback Original

Copyright © 2007 by LaDawn Black

Published in the United States by One World Books,
an imprint of The Random House Publishing Group,
a division of Random House, Inc., New York.

ONE WORLD is a registered trademark and the One World colophon
is a trademark of Random House, Inc.

ISBN 978-0-345-48664-6

Library of Congress Cataloging-in-Publication Data

Black, LaDawn.
Let's get it on : 15 hot tips and tricks to spice up your sex life / by
LaDawn Black.
p. cm.
ISBN 978-0-345-48664-6
1. Sex instruction for women. 2. Sexual excitement. 3. African American
women—Sexual behavior. 4. Man–woman relationships. I. Title.

HQ46.B573 2007
613.9'6—dc22   2006050741

Printed in the United States of America

www.oneworldbooks.net

24687531

Book design by Susan Turner

To the two JBs for love, light, and laughter

Acknowledgments

Thanks can go on forever, so I will try to make this one short and sweet!

I would like to thank my publishing team, V. Sanders, M. Guy, and S. Evans for supporting book one, *Stripped Bare,* and keeping me on track with book two. I could not have done this without you. Thanks also go out to my 92Q family and *blackmeninamerica.com* for promoting my books and providing me with a larger platform for getting the message of good loving out to the masses. Thanks to all of the bookselling, radio, television, and newspaper outlets that have shown their support. As always, thanks to Karibu bookstore for continuing to be an outlet for my work and keeping me plugged into the local literary scene.

Personally, I would like to, as always, acknowledge my very best black men, JB and Alec. Thanks for the love and encouragement as our lives continue to evolve. Love goes out to my core family, the Wrays—Deb and the two Lamonts, thanks for always being there. Thanks to the muse for bringing me passion when I needed it most. Finally, I would like to thank the world's best listeners and readers. I am so encouraged by the way you share your lives with me every day. I know that you look to me for advice, but know that I have learned so much from each of you and I carry you with me.

Peace & Love Always,
—L

Contents

Let's Get
It On

Are You Getting It On?
The Overview

*I am the sexiest sister on the planet. Every day I blow
at least one man's mind by just saying "hello." People
are drawn to me, and my opinion and thoughts
count. Sexually I am a beast, because I do what I
know well and can pick up fast on the new. I am cap-
tivating, engaging, diverse, and open. I am the ultimate hottie dipped in toffee.*

As the host of a number-1 radio show, "The Love
Zone," I am often asked questions about dating,
sex, and relationships both on the air and off. But
when I traveled to promote my first book, *Stripped Bare: The 12
Truths That Will Help You Land the Very Best Black Man*, the
one question that sisters would pose time and time again was
"How can I be more desirable?" I've learned to own my sexuality and use it to project power and strength while putting others at ease, and I want to show you how to do the same. The
paragraph above isn't meant to blow my own horn; it is meant

to show where I am now on a daily basis in my thoughts, attitudes, and deeds, and where you could be by the end of this book.

So many beautiful, intelligent, and successful sisters are still plagued by the idea that they can't be both sexy and respected. They see the images of sexy women in film, music videos, magazines, and movies and rarely see that sexiness balanced with brains. Some sisters fear they will have to dumb themselves down in order to be sexy. But true sexiness isn't about six-pack abs and nutcracker thighs. It doesn't involve being stupid or self-absorbed. Truly sexy people know how to work their magic in such a way that others are encouraged and inspired by it and not put off by their power. Being sexy will unlock all of your best attributes and not force you to down-shift your morals, goals, or ideas.

It is my hope that, after reading this book, you will own your sexuality and have the power to up the ante in pleasure and satisfaction for both yourself and your partner. Sex should be fun and freaky, and I am going to get you to the point where you stop dreaming about the ultimate sexual experience and actually go out and live it. This book will:

- Free you from conventional thoughts on sexual right and wrong
- Show you how to leave your lover wanting more
- School you on keeping a long-term relationship sexy
- Expose you to new sexual techniques that guarantee pleasure
- Let you be the freak that you desire to be

But this book isn't just about having great sex. Taking responsibility for your sexuality will help to increase your self-confidence in all social arenas: family, career, friends, and much more. People who are truly sexy ooze it in every situation every day, and they often forget that they even have the gift. There is something to be said for those individuals who can walk into a room and always be the center of attention. We have all seen the sister who dresses her butt off, is a great conversationalist, and gives off the vibe that you just have to get to know her. We have all met that brother who leaves behind a sense of wonder and amazement when he exits a group. In both cases, the crowd wants to know how they can get some of that.

Each chapter is laid out as follows:

- **My Personal Path Toward Discovery** *All about how I discovered this tip.*

- **Sexy How-To** *Hands-on advice for making the tip work.*

- **Your Result** *The end game of putting the sex tip to work.*

- **Sexual Toolbox** *An additional spicy trick just for you!*

As an added bonus, there are five "soft-core" sex tips sprinkled throughout the book that focus on getting your mind ready for sex. All true sexual divas know that great sex must start in the mind!

Feel free to make notes, laugh, and yell at the book as I teach you a new way of being that doesn't revolve around cosmetics, the gym, hair weaves, or how good your stuff is! I hope that you will see yourself in my own personal stories, as well as those of my friends, my listeners, and my readers, that illustrate the tips throughout the book.

And now my sisters: Let's get it on!

—L

1

Flips and Tricks
Being the Sexual Annihilator

YOUR QUESTION

LaDawn:
I listen to your show every night and it seems that there are so many people out there who are more sexually advanced than I am. I thought that when a sister started doing oral she was really doing something, but the other night other sisters were calling in about threesomes, anal, and tossing salad, and once again I felt behind the curve. Are people really doing these things, or is this just fodder to get on the air?

Sis,
Trust me, they are doing those things and much more!

So many sex guides point to "thinking" that you are sexy as the only criteria for actually being sexy. Not true, all of the mental sexiness in the world will just melt away if you can't back it up with old-fashioned hands-on sexual skill. I want you to slay your partner and leave him wanting more. There are some keys to being the sexual annihilator and both getting the pleasure that you want and pleasing your partner. It's time to get your hands and every other body part into the game and learn the path toward your ultimate pleasure.

My Personal Path Toward Discovery

What do you have in your sexual toolbox? Here are my top five for any sister looking to turn a brother out:

- Something lickable and sweet (cream/gel)
- A medium-sized vibrator to share
- Cuffs or a scarf
- A wig
- Imagination or a great sex guide (like this one!)

Ladies, it is time to get your sex thing on. Think you already know how to do it? Don't think you need a refresher course? Stop kidding yourself, sister—your sex game can always use a jump-start. It is oh so sexy to have someone not only talk the game, but also play it extremely well. A sister who can hold her own sexually never has to brag about it or flaunt it. Men can sense, smell, and even taste good loving before they even get close enough to test it. I am going to walk you through the ways to gain sexual advantage. You will have everyone wanting more.

At some point in life, you figure out where everything goes

and the best ways to make it feel pretty good and get the deed done. I call this teen sex, in that you are satisfied to just be there and have all the equipment do what it is supposed to do. I was in this cycle for a few years, until I came across this brother who unlocked the door to my real sexuality. He gave me tricks and experiences that blew my mind and allowed me to do what I wanted to do with no apologies. We made love everywhere and in every way: on the conference table at his job, on a penthouse balcony, on airplanes, and in some other places that I will take to my grave. But it wasn't just *where* we had sex, it is what we actually did. He taught me all the areas on my body that were sensitive, and he took the time to really show and tell me the many ways to turn him on. I remember to this day his famous quote, "Stop guessing and ask for what you want!"

Now, I am not saying that this brother taught me sex and that this is what you need. What I am really saying is that he taught me to control my own sexuality and to revel in all the pleasure it could give without apologies. After him, I was always looking for the next high, and to this day, even as a married woman, I like to push the envelope. What can I do that is new? Where can we go? How does this feel? It is a constant quest that I hope will continue until I leave this planet.

When I decided to

LET'S GET IT ON TIP 1

Be the Sexual Annihilator

Give yourself a sexual jump-start. Learn something new and implement it.

control my sexual satisfaction, I was better able to convey what I wanted to lovers and be comfortable in my skin. I know what turns me on, and I have a good idea of what turns others on. I can speak confidently about sex, and my lover knows he can bring anything to me and we can try it out. Hotties know the power of true sex appeal. It heats up on your skin and works itself through the room, letting others know that you can handle yours. Are you giving off your best sexual vibe?

Sexy How-To

Sex is a muscle that needs to be worked and researched, like any other leisure activity that you want to stay on top of. Don't get locked into the 1-2-3 of sex and just assume that because orgasm is reached, that is enough. There should always be passion, experimentation, discovery, and fun when it comes to sex, and if you have been missing those elements for some time, you may need to be doing something else.

There truly is an inner glow that radiates from within when the sex thing is clicking. Sex can improve your health and mental outlook. There are definite benefits for keeping it interesting and active. Dust the guides off and bring out the toys, because you need to get your sex thing on lock.

Follow these three points to sexual beast territory:

RESEARCH . . . RESEARCH . . . RESEARCH.
Study the latest sexual techniques, trends, and buzz words. Try to incorporate as many of the tricks as possible into your love play. Ask others what they find sexy, and get feedback on what

works and what doesn't. Sexy conversation is always a great icebreaker.

Dress it up.

Put the cotton undergarments away for a month. Lose the comfy sack PJs and college sweats and tees. For one month, go all-out sexy even when you are alone. Great body lotions, treatments, and scents should be added to the mix. Sometimes the easiest way to experience a rebirth is to actually start to feel it from the outside in.

Have a purely sexual encounter.

If you are already linked or if you have a friend with benefits, why not take your lover on a purely sexual romp? Tell him that making love is out of the window and the session tonight is all about fucking and the many ways to do it. I know it may shock his system, but this is a great method to try out your new sexual self in a nonthreatening way because you are being the sexual diva tonight and not the same old Diane.

Your Result

Bringing the heat sexually allows you to reinforce all of the outer sexy signs with a little passion secret within that says to the world "You don't know everything about me." Plus who can overlook all of the mental and physical benefits of being sexually on? People who are sexually satisfied look better, are more self-confident, and simply radiate confidence with the opposite sex because they know that they can take on whatever another has to dish out.

Sexual Toolbox

Develop a "let's talk about it" approach to sex with your partner. Share on a daily basis the craziest news stories, TV or
movie clips, or conversation of the day of a sexual tone. Ask for
opinions and thoughts and pay attention, because while you
may not be specifically discussing your relationship, your partner may be telling you a great deal about his desires, wants,
and needs in the bedroom.

2

Loving the Opposite
Really Liking Men

LaDawn,
Look, I know you are so pro-brother. I read the first
book and you just give them a pass in saying that sis-
ters are the problem when it comes to relationships. I
totally disagree. Brothers are cruddy these days. They
will run all over and use you and throw you back
when they are done. I am so fed up that I swear at
times I think that maybe I'd be happier if I became a
lesbian. Stop letting the brothers off and face the fact
that a lot of them are indeed bad and unfit and a lot of
sisters are going to be alone.

Sister:
I never give bad brothers a pass, and I have been
around the relationship wheel enough to know that
yes, there are some brothers out there that need to
work on their shit before ever even breathing on a
woman. Honestly, however, I stand by my principle
that most of our problems with relationships are our
own fault. Like in your letter, you seem very negative
on brothers and not willing to take a chance. Do you

really think brothers aren't sensing this when you come around? I am not asking you to turn into a fool or to fall for all of the games, but I do think an attitude adjustment is needed if you ever hope to actually have a man feel wanted or appreciated in your presence.

P.S. The whole lesbian thing may not be the answer for you either, because there are some bad women out there too! Then what will you turn to—monkeys? Keep the faith, sister.

*T*his is my favorite!!!!!
     I am getting ready to piss a few sisters off now, because this Getting It On tip is all about loving the brothers. Any brother will tell you that the sexiest and most appealing women are those that really get and like men. A lot of us deal with men, but we secretly don't trust or like them. Do you think men don't pick up on this? They can clearly make the distinction between women who really want them and those who merely see them as a means to an end (kids, stability, financial gain, etc.).

This tip is my favorite because it is one that I did not have to do a great deal of study on. I love men. I always have, and I get such a kick out of their energy, style, and view of the world. I am not just a fan of one type of brother—I love them all, and that love speaks volumes about how men view me on a daily basis. Women who like men are not only seen as being sexy, they are also viewed as being part of the team. If you really like them, they want you around all the time, and you can never, ever lose when one of them is in your corner.

You want to be the ultimate woman for any man—so sister, you'd better start liking them!

My Personal Path Toward Discovery

Long ago I knew that my attraction first to boys and then to men was strong. I am not just talking in a sexual sense. I enjoy hanging with my girls, but time with my male friends has always been a little more wonderful. Spending time with the opposite sex really gives you a look into a totally different world of how men think, what they do, what they think is important, and honestly what they think about women. This knowledge is priceless.

In liking men I have been able to move through career circles easily, navigate social scenes, and learn the fine art of interpreting male behavior and thought. Unlike most women, my love of men is diverse: I love all races, sizes, and age groups. I have learned just as much from a sixty-year-old divorcé as I did from a twenty-one-year-old college student. These friendships have enriched my life and made me a well-rounded woman.

As I do seminars around the country, so many women want a man in their lives, but when they get into their experiences with men it becomes clear that they want someone in their lives that they have not taken the time to study and get to know. You can't just pick up a man like a pair of shoes. You have to understand what he likes, what you want, and whether or not he is going to be a good fit. Liking men will do wonders for your study, because guys will tell a woman everything if she appears to not be on a search for anything.

I am going to show you how truly liking men can boost your sexual temperature, because while you can indeed win them over with a tight mental game, the game has to be appreciative and respectful of maleness.

LET'S GET IT ON TIP 2

Start to Really Like Men

Work on getting to know and really appreciate brothers. When you enter into their world you can share their secrets with the rest of us, and how hot is that?

Sexy How-To

I was doing a relationship seminar recently and a sister posed this question: "How can I get my man to tell me what he really wants?" This sister was trying to please her man, but was having a really hard time making things come together. She didn't feel that he was being totally honest about his sexual desires, and she was getting tired of playing the guessing game.

My advice to this sister was to create an environment where her man would not feel judged when it came to his sexual needs. Is she playful and sexual outside of the bedroom? Does she inquire in nonsexual situations about movie sex scenes, sexy clothing, or magazine covers to gauge his level of interest? Is she letting her man know that she is open to all of his fantasies? These are the ways to get a man to be up-front with you about his turn-ons. Your girls can't tell you what your man wants, and no relationship expert can give you the full picture either. Ask your man in nonthreatening and fun ways and you will get the answer that you are seeking. Where did I get this insight? From male friends who felt comfortable enough around me to tell me the truth.

Liking men is a skill that all women should have, but very few possess. Have you sat and actually listened to how most women talk about men? They describe them as dogs, buffoons, selfish, egotistical—and I could go on and on. Most women desire a man only so they can say that they have one, not because he brings anything special or unique to her life. Since women have often been hurt or disappointed by men in the past, most just decide it is best not to get too involved and have little or no time for any man.

Wrong! Wrong! Wrong! Tip number two is key to developing sexy status. Loving the opposite sex (this is true for the brothers as well) makes you golden because you are able to move around freely in enemy territory with an all-access pass. When you let men know that you really like them, they start to pass the message around to their friends that X is the hottest woman around because she gets us—she is chill. Being chill gets you info, attention, and great male references. I am not blowing smoke here. So many of my best hook-ups and opportunities, both personal and professional, have come from great brothers just looking to help a sister out. Believe me, these brothers don't do this for every sister—only the sisters that make them feel comfortable and appreciated.

The Male Map

Here is your map to a man's pleasure points. Don't just think penis, nipples, and balls. There is so much more on the male frame to play with and tantalize. Here are ten key body parts to keep on your radar in any intimate situation:

1. THE BRAIN

Do not downplay the role of mental stimulation in creating an ideal sexual scenario. Seduce all day long and use many different tools. Enlist e-mail, text messages, photos, and voice messages as seduction tools. Let your man know over breakfast what you plan on doing to him later in the day. Instead of always looking forward to "making love," try "fucking" him instead. Let him know while you are fucking him how you like it and what you want next. Sex his brain and he will be yours.

2. TOES

We often overlook a brother's toes as a point of passion entry. Honestly, there are brothers out there with crusty feet that we feel it's best to ignore. Why not surprise your man by giving him the foot stimulation that he craves? You can treat him to a pedicure at a spa or give him one at home. Once his feet are straight, sisters, it's time for a foot rub, some licking, and even a little toe sucking. The toes kind of flow with everything below the belt as tension zones and ultimate pleasure points. Another suggestion: The next time you are on top during intercourse, turn around and face his feet. Lean over and rub his feet as you ride him. I promise you that this will be a ride he will not quickly forget.

3. BEHIND THE KNEES

Most men are sensitive both behind their knees and down along their calves. These are prime foreplay areas where a great massage or quick lick would be appreciated. As you take the body tour, why not get your man on his belly and rub the back of his legs? For a bit of extra punch, add some warming oil to the equation so that with each breath and lick he gets a warm sensation.

4. THE ANAL AREA

This one is always fun because most sisters are scared to step to a brother's butt. There are two main reasons for this: most brothers cinch up at the mere thought of anal play, and because of all the hair, most sisters aren't sure what awaits them at the end of the brick road. Now, let's say you have overcome a brother's fear and hygiene and you want to play. Here is your game plan: True anal play begins with a butt massage. Next, add kisses to the cheeks and light licks, slowly lick the outside of the anus, and then add a twist by inserting your tongue. Warning: If the brother loves the tongue, he may be open to a finger or a small toy. Don't be amazed; many straight men are turned on by anal play, and sisters, if you haven't been turned out anally, you are missing a treat as well.

5. INSIDE/UNDER THE ARMS

Okay, we all like to hold hands while having sex—this is often one of the most wonderful ways to feel connected to your lover. The next time you grab his hands during intercourse or while going down on him, run your fingers down the underside of his arms, and even through his armpits. Armpits are under-appreciated for their sensitive nature, and brothers often miss out on armpit titillation because of the hair that blocks the area. You can start with your fingertips, maybe even use your tongue, but the money move is to run your nipples along the underside of his arms and even along the armpits. The hair will give you a bit of a tingle as well.

6. Top of the Head

You have to do head worship. If his head is bald or cut low, it is so easy to just lick and kiss the top of his head while kissing his face, licking his ears, or allowing him to suck your breasts. If the brother has dreads or an Afro, then you should focus on kissing the forehead while massaging his scalp with your fingertips. The scalp is full of nerve endings that deserve to be put to work. Next time you are loving his face, make sure that you don't forget that there is another head worthy of your mouth.

7. Lower Back above the Butt

Just as we like to have the small of our back kissed and massaged, so do brothers. The crevice right above their butt is a prime area for your fingers, lips, and toes. You can add a little oil and feathers or a silk scarf for an extra tease. The sensitivity is incredible in this area, and the whole time you are playing, he is wondering how far down you plan on going. For an extra surprise while licking his lower back, why not go all the way down and give his balls a lick from behind? It will be a huge surprise that will pay off in more surprises for you.

8. Stomach

Oftentimes the male stomach is overlooked because the contour and softness of a lady's stomach is held in such high regard. The truth is that a brother with killer abs is just as hot as a sister with perfect form, and their abs deserve some love as well. You can go the typical route of kisses and fingertips, but the ultimate turn-on for most men is for you to run your body and hair along their stomach. Start kissing his face and slowly snake your body along his. Men love this "accidental" brushing of your body against their skin. This is also a great move for your man's back.

9. Back of the Neck

There is nothing more sexy than a kiss in an unexpected place. Instead of focusing on the lips only, why not take your best lip game to the brother's neck: but make it the back of the neck. The back-of-the-neck kiss can be sensuous and unexpected. Also, it provides access to the back of the ears and shoulder blades—areas that are often overlooked as hot zones. To add to the heat factor, try writing a sexy message on the back of his neck with a ballpoint pen or using body paint to create a sexy image or note.

10. Fingers

A brother's fingers are super-sensitive during sex. There is so much that you can do to and with his fingers to make the sex incredible. You can of course suck them, but the sexiest thing you can do is place his fingers on your body and softly tell him what to do once you've placed them there. Brothers love when you position their hands during most sexual acts. Show him when and how to grab your butt during intercourse; show him how to touch your breasts or what to touch when he goes down on you. Another thing to try is the next time he is touching himself, make sure you kiss and lick his fingers to help

him out and demonstrate how turned on you are by seeing
him get himself off.

Your Result

In order for liking men to really work for you, you have to understand this main point: Liking men does not mean sexing all
of them. It means that all of your interactions with men
throughout the day, from your man to the grocery guy to Steve
in the mailroom, are tinged with a bit of play that shows them
that you appreciate them. For some women this takes the form
of a smile and how ya' do, and for others it is as simple as just
changing their internal perception of men—they are not the
enemy, and they can indeed be an asset.

I would suggest that you start with any male friends that
you already have. Ask them about how you come off and what
you can do to be more approachable. No male friends? (How
sad!) Then try some male relatives. Start working on their suggestions and get out and mingle. Personally, I think the best
way to bring any man into your fold is eye contact, touch, and
listening. Being present goes a long way toward making people
feel that you're special.

On the sexual side, you have to know that men are unique
in their sexual desires. Take the time to ask what turns them
on and truly be open to doing whatever it takes. Prepare yourself for the strange requests (keep your white cotton panties
on during intercourse all the time was an actual request from
one of my more spaced-out lovers) to the fairly routine (role-
playing and talking dirty). Don't get offended or run for the
hills, because this is a dialogue that will unlock the key to

being the special sister who does it all for him that he will never, ever want to lose.

Sexual Toolbox

Take the "Chatty Cathy Challenge": For one full week, speak to every man that passes your way. A simple hello can spark conversation with great brothers looking to get to know a great sister. Just think of all the brothers you may have missed out on by being defensive or keeping your head buried in the newspaper or your eyes glued to the computer screen. Be a "Chatty Cathy" and see how much of a difference it makes in expanding your man pool.

3

So Smooth

Personal Care

YOUR QUESTION

LaDawn,
In response to your question about craziest sexual re-
quests ever, my man wants me to shave his initials into
my pubic hair.

Sister:
There are waxers and waxing kits out there that can
give your man the pubic hair adoration that he desires
from you, but just for fun, ask him if he is willing to
return the favor on his chest, head, or butt. I'm guessing no, but let me know what he says.

*T*ouch really drives the sexual experience. Think
about how, when the lights are low or off and you
are feeling your man, you connect to him by just
the feel of his skin, the texture of his hair, and the hardness of
his body. He enjoys you in the very same way, often tracing the

beauty of your body with his hands before tasting you with his tongue or entering you with his penis.

It is important to make sure that all of you is desirable to him. Tip number three goes beyond the dressing to the best ways to feel, taste, and smell better. So Smooth is all about getting your body up to snuff so that you feel sexually confident and he wants to explore it in every way imaginable.

My Personal Path Toward Discovery

A lover in my past really encouraged me to experience his body. It was easy to appraise and enjoy what I saw, but what would happen if I simply closed my eyes and explored? This brother would not only ask how something felt, he would ask how it tasted and smelled. In return, he told me what he experienced with me. It was the first time that I had a brother describe my hips as buttery and warm and my boobs as engrossing and honey-like. Let's just say that a sister was hooked, and I wanted more. Also, this brother taught me that sex during the day or with the lights on can be ridiculously sexy. There is nothing to hide, and you can accentuate the visual with the other senses. Sex can be crazy with that level of sensory stimulation.

This brother showed

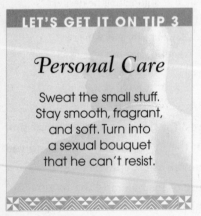

LET'S GET IT ON TIP 3

Personal Care

Sweat the small stuff.
Stay smooth, fragrant,
and soft. Turn into
a sexual bouquet
that he can't resist.

me that sex is more than just putting things in the right places—it is also about all of the unique qualities that we bring to the table. This brother loved smooth skin, so a sister learned real quick to shave and wax everywhere. I felt free enough to let him know that I love hair on a man, so he let his hair grow on his chest and head, and it was so sexy. We played with our favorite scents and took pleasure in the way our love-making enhanced them. Sex turned into a sensory game with high stakes.

Sexy How-To

Sisters at times seem confused when it comes to present-ing their ideal sexual selves without clothes. Should you shave or not? What is the perfect scent? Is there any way to improve your vaginal taste and scent? Like most things in life, these things are very subjective, because some brothers love hairy legs while others run from the very hint of body hair. Some brothers love perfume while others like to bask in the natural scent of you. At times it seems hard to figure it all out.

The real answer to these types of questions is that you must first determine what you are most comfortable with and what you can maintain and then ask your man what he prefers. The point of this particular truth is that it is important to be just as concerned with your naked sexiness as you are with the outside-world sexiness of clothes and makeup.

Here are the areas that can help you step up your sexual game when it comes to improving your personal care:

SHAVING

There are men who like their women smooth everywhere. That means, sisters, you need to be up on the latest waxing, shaving, and sugaring techniques. There are even permanent laser solutions to get rid of the hair. Also, note that I am not just talking underarms and legs here, ladies. Today it is preferred by most to have the vagina shaved, waxed, or neatly trimmed—bushes rarely appeal. Anal areas should not be neglected. If you like to get your back-door thing on, why not try a Brazilian wax that hits the anal area and maybe even an anal bleaching to lighten the area? Brothers tell me all the time that a well-maintained vagina is more appealing and allows for easier access to everything.

EXFOLIATING

Get your skin in shape, sisters. Invest in a great exfoliant to smooth everything out and make your skin feel like butter. Using an exfoliant will not only make the skin texture feel smoother, but in many cases it can reduce the appearance of cellulite. There are so many formulas at your local drugstore that will give you back that baby-soft skin and smooth out all of your rough edges.

TASTE

Look into all-natural products when it comes to lotions and scents. Try to get products that taste as good as they make you feel. There are products at your grocery store that can be used as moisturizers and lubricants that are functional and taste great. Here are some items that can be mashed or spread on the skin that have beauty benefits and add sexual intrigue: strawberries, honey, papaya, peaches, and yogurt.

There are also sexual potions that taste great and provide a sexual function. Visit your local adult novelty store or go online for the latest in warming creams, body mousse, flavored lubricants, and much more.

SMELL

Be wild when it comes to your scents. Apply scents to your skin and hair that are exotic and off the beaten path. Stay away from popular scents and learn how to layer natural essential oils in order to have your own signature scent.

Stop covering up your natural vaginal scent with sprays and washes. Most men are turned on by the natural scent of a woman, and if you are physically healthy and treating your body right, your natural scent should not be at all offensive.

TOUCH FACTOR

Make sure that you are moisturizing your skin daily. It is so easy to make sure that your soap, shampoo, and lotions are all working together. The quality and feel of your skin is important to your overall sexiness in that skin condition often is the first indicator of physical health, personal upkeep, and overall hygiene level.

Your Result

Paying close attention to how you care for your body will allow you to not only look seductive, but literally feel it. Brothers tell me all the time that women lose sexy points based on the little things: cracked feet, lack of shaving, chapped lips, and much more. Why not take care of yourself better just for you first? You will be shocked by how much glistening skin and a great scent will add to your overall sex appeal.

Sexual Toolbox

Instead of always shaving yourself, why not have the man in your life do it for you? Most men are turned on by the intimacy and strange excitement in engaging in your personal ritual. You can let him do the legs, but if you want a four-star evening, let him shave your vagina as well.

SOFT-CORE SEX TIP #1
Boost Your Sense of You

Why is it so wrong to think that you are sexy? To admit to yourself and the world that you are the finest, smartest, and most desirable thing ever? Ladies, if we don't think we are fabulous, then no one will. To be a real sexual diva, you need a great deal of self-esteem and confidence. You have to ooze the stuff. There is a fine art to having the highest level of confidence and showing it while not putting people off. Think it is impossible to do? Let me show you.

Sexy How-To

Being confident in yourself is really a gift that you should give to your spirit every day. There is so much in the world that can make us feel inadequate, so it is crucial that we build up emotional and physical armor to fend off personal attacks.

You need to come up with a way to remind yourself daily how great you are. Many sisters that I have worked with on this have used daily planners, notes on the refrigerator, and even screen savers at work to reinforce their positive traits. Once you have these ingrained in your mind, you will find that you walk a little straighter, negotiate better, and network more effectively, among other benefits. If you believe in your greatness, it can't help but radiate.

But be warned—extreme self-esteem sometimes comes with a price. You have to know how to balance it with humility. When you are extremely confident, some may see you as arrogant. It is important that you learn when and how to exercise your confidence. Complimenting others and showing an interest in them are two ways to balance out your new super-confident self with some softer points to make others more comfortable with your new sexy diva status.

4

Follow the Leader

Ask Him What He Wants

LaDawn,
Are all men turned on by the same things? I suggested
watching porn with my new man and he looked at me
as if I'd suggested sex with a baby pig. Other men have
been turned on by this idea. Why is my man so turned
off by porn?

Sister:
What is sexy for one brother may not be sexy for all.
Make sure that when you meet someone new, you
take the time to get to know what turns that particular brother on. You won't win anyone over giving the
same old stuff—each man is unique in his passion
tastes. Get to know his by asking.

With most things in life, we take the time to get to
know new situations, people, and things. You
meet someone new on the job and take her out
to lunch to get to know her better. You buy a new car and read

the manual to see how all of its features work. You even take the time to get acquainted with the best ways to operate your new flat-panel television. It is amazing to me how often we do not take the time to get to know or learn to operate a new man.

We women think we have it all figured out when it comes to men. We think we know how they expect us to look, act, and smell. We think there is a certain routine to making love, and all relationships progress from casual dating to serious relationship and on to engagement within 2.5 years. Yep, we have it all figured out without even once asking the brother a question.

Sex is no different, in that we often assume that all guys want and like the same thing. News flash, ladies: Brothers are just as diverse in their appetites as we are. What works for one does not work for all. The easiest way to know how to best turn your man on is to simply ask him.

My Personal Path Toward Discovery

Okay, I was spoiled by one brother. He introduced me to the concept of having sex in public. We would do it on rooftops overlooking the city, on the side of the road, at beaches and parks—basically anywhere that we could stop long enough to get everything up and ready. One time we actually made love in the conference room at his job that had an incredible view of D.C. at night. To this day I remember how exciting and beautiful that was, along with the distinct chill of the marble tabletop. This brother could not get enough of the threat of being discovered when it came to where we were together. Once we even found ourselves in the telephone closet of a hotel because we couldn't make it up to our room. Even after this relationship ended, I came across other brothers who shared this urge to push the limits.

Then a new brother came along who was definitely sensual, so why not see what we could get going. On several occasions I suggested that we just drop trou and get busy

where we were instead of trying to get back to his place or mine. After about the third suggestion, I finally caught on to the idea that this brother was not interested in public sex. Finally, after being quite confused for some time, I asked him about whether or not public displays were for him. What I found out was that this brother felt that we could have a serious relationship and he believed that if he treated me like a trick, I would be a trick for him. So he wanted to keep our relationship as traditional as possible in an effort to keep it special. Now, personally, I don't think that public sex means that you are loose, but the brother had a right to his own opinion. By asking the question, I was able to better gauge what turned him on and make peace with things that turned him off. Sisters, we just have to ask the question to find out what he desires instead of assuming that we know.

Sexy How-To

There are many ways to take your man's temperature when it comes to what turns him on sexually. Some women are comfortable just asking the question, while other sisters search out subtle ways to get the intel that they need. There are many ways to find out what your man wants and put plans into place to please him the way that he desires to be pleased.

- Ask him what worked for him in the past. Have him share his greatest and worst sexual experiences with you.

- Inquire about the women he thinks are sexy. Note the types of women that appeal to him. If all of the women he names are classy and ladylike, then maybe the thugged-out chick style isn't for him.

- Ask his opinion about particular scenes in regular or adult movies. This is for the shy sister. While watching a movie, ask your man what he thought of a particularly sexy scene. From his answer, you should be able to determine his level of kink.

- Ask, "What do you enjoy about us being together? What do you wish was different?" I call this the self-evaluation. This isn't just for a new relationship. Ask the brother this throughout the relationship to make sure he is being pleased. Flip it on him for your satisfaction as well.

- Ask, "What is your greatest fantasy?" This really gets to the heart of your greatest desires and what you like to do. Be prepared, however, for strange offerings—one brother told me that his greatest fantasy was to whip me until I bled and then lick the blood off. Luckily, I got out of this one right at the kissing stage!

- Get the clues. If you are not the questioning type, then simply observe your man. What does he enjoy that you do to him? What does he turn away from or not act on? Are there turn-ons that he shares with you without being prompted? Do the investigative work to piece together his erotic map.

Your Result

In most things in life, we seek out an expert before jumping in and getting the job done. Why in the world do we just assume that we already know what a man may want? Take advantage of the opportunity to ask and observe your man's passion accelerators. Stop the guessing game and you will automatically tighten up your sexual game, because you are hitting home runs every time.

The other plus of this approach is that you are inspiring your man to ask you the very same questions. You are creating an environment where sexual communication and the exchange of ideas are welcome. Finally, you will have a man in your life who is interested in new ways to please you and not simply hoping to get it right.

Sexual Toolbox

Not ready to have heavy sexual discussions quite yet? Why not take a tour around his body? One night, just go from body part to body part licking, tickling, and rubbing your way to discovering his sexy spots. I tried this one night and discovered the wild heat of belly buttons. Who knew!!

5
A Kid at Heart
Games

LaDawn,

I find playing stranger games really stupid. Most relationship guides suggest meeting your partner out in public and acting like you don't know each other and the sparks are suppose to just start. I tried this with my husband and it didn't work, because how do you act like you don't know a person who has been with you for over a decade? Is there a game out there that can be sexy and make sense?

P.S. No schoolgirl outfits either—something is just inherently wrong about that.

Sister:

There are so many sexual games out there for adults that involve a whole bunch of planning and costumes. One of my favorites is playing naked scavenger hunt around your home. Send the kids away and place notes around and even outside of the home to send your man on the search for you, or maybe for something the two of you have been wanting to experience (a new sex toy or video, for example). Have fun with it and make the clues sexy.

The truth is that any traditional game can become sexual—just strip down and add whipped cream. Enjoy!

One of the simplest ways to make sex fun is to add a game or two to the mix. Many of us played quite a bit of strip poker in college, or perhaps truth or dare, but it's time to play more adult games for higher stakes. When was the last time that you planned a night of games? Have you lost your interest in sexual play? When you start dating someone, you are constantly planning what is going to be different about the next interlude. Maybe you even roll out all of the sexual tools that seem to drive men crazy (vibrators, ticklers, and other such devices). But often, once a relationship is established, we roll our sense of play out the door in favor of comfortable sex.

Then there is the sister who has absolutely no play in her whatsoever. It doesn't present itself in new relationships and it never is discovered as a relationship matures. Does this sister really believe that sex can't be playful? Does she realize how much she is missing by not laughing in bed?

I am going to free my sourpusses and former gamers from their inhibitions. You should play in bed, because sometimes getting there (foreplay) can be more fulfilling than the main event (intercourse).

My Personal Path Toward Discovery

I love to laugh in bed. Trying something new and getting it all wrong is sometimes one of the sexiest moments you can share with a person. Playing games shows that you want to be engaged when it comes to sex and not just lie there.

One of my favorite gamers was a boyfriend from college. He was an art major, and he was amazing. One night when we were together, I asked him to draw something for me. Now I know that this brother has probably drawn for a lot of sisters, but I asked him to literally draw *on* me. The game I came up with was for him to draw on my various body parts what he liked and how they made him feel and to come up with a creative way to link all of the areas.

The brother definitely thought I had lost my mind, but he got his markers out and went to work. The sensuality that was generated in his room that night was incredible, with the pen feeling like a feather on my skin and his breath warming me as he tried to quickly dry the

> **LET'S GET IT ON TIP 5**
>
> ## *Get in the Game*
>
> Add a sense of play to your sexual activity. You will uncover surprising talents and interests of your lover while breaking the missionary mode.

ink. By the end, we were so busy laughing and critiquing the work that we nearly woke up his roommate sleeping only a few feet away (don't act like you didn't have sex with a roommate in the room back in the day).

Instead of simply washing his art off in the morning, we

photographed it. All these years later I still have the photos. What a sexy game to play, and what a great memory we created!

Sexy How-To

Not feeling too creative? Here are some suggestions:

- Turn any traditional board game into a naked version. This isn't too hard—just suggest that the next time you plan to crush him in checkers that he not have anything on.

- Serve your next meal nude and in heels. Let him know that he cannot touch you until the meal is complete.

- Be his sexy video girl. Allow him to shoot nude photos/videos of you. Let him direct and pick poses. Just make sure you have in your possession the only copy of any photos/videos when the session is over!

- Let him eat his favorite dessert off of you. Or place his favorite drink on your body for him to indulge in.

- Play naked Twister.

The super-creative sister may want to try these:

- Create a whole different sexual persona. Give yourself a name, a wig, and an accent, and please him in ways that he has not yet thought of. Maybe even invite another woman into the mix for variety.

- Most women have done a striptease for their man, but why not dance at a real club only for him? You can rent the space or go at an off-time for a local club. What a turn-on for him to actually see you perform!

- Film your next sexual tryst without letting him know, or capture yourself alone and send the video to his phone. A quick six-second video will get him to hurry home for more video fun.

- Spend one night having sex using only your mouth—no hands or toys allowed.

- Create a personal website where only he has the URL. Install a webcam that allows him to see you in your most intimate moments at any point during the day. He can do the same, and the two of you can have fun being voyeurs all day long.

Your Result

The truth is that sex can, like most things in the world, become very routine if the partners are no longer actively engaged. Games and a sense of play keep sexual activity light and fun. By incorporating play into your amour, you are letting a person know that you are interested in keeping things interesting. Also, sexual play is a key indicator as to whether or not someone is a good lover. Often the best lovers in the world are the ones who are not afraid to try something new and laugh while trying to pull it off.

Sexual Toolbox

Your bedroom should have the following items close at hand for any type of sexual play: dice, cuffs, massage cream, paper, markers, paint and paintbrush, and a candle. All of these items can be great props for turning any traditional game into a sexual one.

6
Lickity Stix
Perfecting Your Oral Form

LaDawn,
Does a man like his anus licked when a woman is going down on him? I know I like when my man goes there, but most straight men are strange when it comes to that. Should I try it or leave it alone?

Sister:
I suggest you walk carefully when it comes to this one. Most women tell me that although their men get comfortable with anal stimulation, that first attempt was a bit shocking for them. You may want to start slow with caressing the area between his balls and the anus while he is having an orgasm. Then maybe try a finger in the anus or kissing his butt cheeks. One day, when you feel brave enough, try your tongue. Get ready for the body spasm. Once the sex is over, your man will let you know clearly if he is not interested in reliving that experience. If he appears to enjoy it and puts up no argument, pat yourself on the back, because you have just found another way to get him off.

*I*f you are not getting your blow-job thing on, sister, I feel so sorry for you. One of the most pleasureful things that you can do for yourself is to go down on your man. Note—I did not say the most pleasureful thing that you can do for *him,* because personally, along with a lot of other women, I have found that performing orally perfectly can yield orgasmic results for a woman as well as for a man. You just have to step up your oral skills and learn the many tricks to make it more than just a plain old slob-down.

Ladies, oral sex is no longer an option in most women's sexual menu—it is an entrée. If you want him to joyfully and enthusiastically go down on you, you had better be willing to return the favor. And in this case, the favor isn't simply a quick ball lick and tip kiss. It is really sucking, twisting, and playing with your man's cock to the point where he thinks nothing and no one in the world can get better than this. I'm going to share with you how to big up your blow-job game.

My Personal Path Toward Discovery

I am always looking for better ways to do things. When it comes to sex, I want to know three simple things from any man I have ever been involved with:

What do you like?

What do you wish I would do?

What could I do better?

Now when it comes to oral sex, there is always a bonus question:

What do you want me to do when I go down on you?

Answers have been rather diverse, from giving a soft bite to a little tug, but they never, ever disappoint. I equate the differences in men's preferences in oral sex to our own very distinct opinions on nipple attention. Personally, I am not big on having my nipples played with because they hurt most of the time, while other women consider nipple play crucial to foreplay and one of the main ways to get off. As with men, the touch and technique of oral sex is very individual.

The main thing that I have learned is that all men love it, but you have to be really observant as to how they want it. Some men like to take charge and put you where they want you, while others like to just lie back and let you get the job done. My personal favorite is to have a brother surprise me with what he likes to mix in with his blow job. One brother liked to have his nipples twisted while I was going down (back in my more flexible years), and another introduced me to the fine art of Tantric blow jobs that involve a lot of taking you to the point of the big O and backing off until you are ready for the grand finale (not my favorite, because I think I may have developed a jaw click from this brother).

In the end, it is important to master many different ways to blow. There is so much more to a blow job than a wet mouth, and if you become skilled enough at it, you will start to find your performance as gratifying as does the brother who is receiving it.

LET'S GET IT ON TIP 6

Perfect Your Oral Form

A blow job is more than just lips and a tongue. Giving a top-notch performance involves really putting your back and much more into it.

Sexy How-To

Make your oral skills really stand out by doing more than your average sister. By simply including a few extra moves, you can take your oral play from just adequate to astonishing. Try these tips as starters:

- Be excited about performing the act, and make sure you look up at him while doing it. It works in porn and it can work for you, because it is showing that not only are you sucking him off, but that you are in it only for him.

- Deep throat and twist. My gay friends taught me this trick. It is essential to get as much of the shaft in your mouth as possible and go up and down in a twisting motion. Make sure that when your hands aren't twisting on the shaft, they are gently cupping his balls. All of the motion adds to the friction and sensation of the act.

- Pay extra attention to the balls. Lick, suck, and kiss them along with the inner thighs, belly, and taint (the area under the balls all the way back to the anus). If your man is up for it, insert a finger into his anus or simply lick it for increased pleasure.

- Allow him to please you while you are going down on him. Prop your body up along his so that he can play with or lick you. Better yet, why not have him use your favorite vibe on you while you are going down on him?

- Add a vibe to the oral act. Get a silver bullet and apply it to his balls while you are going down for an extra tingle.

- Make use of the many sexual enhancers on the market that heat up or cool down oral play. There are gels, creams, and powders that heighten orgasms by cooling things down or heating them up. Plus there are many flavors that simply make everything taste great.

- Ask him what he likes when it comes to oral sex. Each man is different, and he may surprise you with his particular oral twist.

Your Result

Step outside of what your girls have taught you about oral sex and experience it on a whole new level. Let go of that old thinking that it is all for him, and open yourself up to the possibility that it can be just as, if not more, satisfying for you. Get away from the simple suck and learn to tantalize new areas on his penis, play with it more, and work in new tricks and potions to heighten the experience. Soon you will be a blow-job pro—not exactly a résumé-builder for the average sister, but it will make all the difference in sexual vitae.

Sexual Toolbox

Chill a pair of ben-wa balls to rub on his balls and stomach while going down on him. Also, invest in a cock ring to prolong his erection and make him extra sensitive to touch.

SOFT-CORE SEX TIP #2
Look the Part

You just can't get away from this—you have to look it. Sisters, stop fooling yourselves. Men are visual when it comes to sex, and if it looks good, they are more apt to partake. There is nothing sinful in showing off a little leg and cleavage on occasion. Also, there is absolutely nothing wrong with being creative and enhancing your natural beauty with additional hair, colored contacts, a plastic surgeon's knife, or makeup, if that is what you want to do. It is all about the fantasy and making you feel your sexy best.

Learn this lesson early! No matter how conservative he is, your man is indeed checking out the latest videos, men's magazines, and that hot sister in accounting. They see and appreciate sexy sisters every day. Don't think that your wholesome beauty is all he needs—every man yearns for the fantasy, and there are more than enough women out there living the fantasy every day to keep him fed. Are you feeding his appetite?

Sexy How-To

ASSESS YOUR SEXINESS.

What is sexy? Evaluate magazines, videos, and films to gather intel on what is considered sexy.

UPDATE YOUR HAIR AND MAKEUP.

Go to the mall and get your makeup professionally done once a year. When it comes to hair, make sure that whatever style you rock is touchable. The most unsexy thing a sister can do is have hair that can't be touched.

BUY LINGERIE FOR YOUR BODY TYPE.

Make sure that all of your lingerie fits well. That means going into a store and having your boobs measured and buying the proper size underwear for your "goddess mounds." Make sure that you have two kinds of lingerie. You should have starter lingerie—functional pieces (supportive, breathable, and comfortable) that are sexy but that you wear every day. Then you have your bench riders—pieces of lingerie that make an appearance only when you are trying to knock his socks off (hint: lots of see-through, lace, push-up, and at times latex).

WEAR SUITS THAT ARE SUGGESTIVE AND POWERFUL.

Make sure your suits are in surprising colors, fit well, and show off a great neckline, strong arms, a tiny waist, or great legs. Lose the hosiery and keep your legs shaved, or switch to the great high-end fishnet hosiery on the market.

WEAR SWEATS THAT TEASE AND DON'T HANG.

If a sweat suit is baggy, throw it away! Ditto any sweat garment with stains or holes, or that you hold on to for multi-use (such as a painting garment). It's time to up the sexy quotient, and just as maternity clothes have become sexy in the new millennium, so have sweats. Make sure that your sweats have a close fit that is flattering to your form. Look at low-slung styles in surprising fabrics. Lose the tee underneath and wear the jacket alone, suggestively unzipped.

WEAR FEEL-GOOD FABRICS.

Become obsessed with how things feel on your skin. Pick clothing that is lush and soft. Look for good stretch and colors that are calming and warming to your skin tones. Get away from black and red as sexy colors and try neutrals, baby blues, or other surprisingly sexy shades.

WEAR HEELS TO DIE FOR.

Stop wearing flat shoes! I know they are comfortable and easy to put on in a pinch, but really, the same way everything looks better by candlelight, all things look tighter, taller, more toned, and tastier in heels. You know I am right, and it's time to just accept the universal truth. Go out and get some heels and I promise you, jeans and a tee can have the same effect as a thong and nipple-out bra. Or at least pretty darn close.

7
Work That Muscle
Exercise to Ecstasy

Hey Girl:
Question: Which do men really prefer, thin women or big-boned girls?

I am full-figured and I have never been without a date, but it seems to me that many brothers want to hide their attraction to me from their boys instead of celebrating it the way they do when we are alone. Why can't men be real with themselves that beauty and sex appeal is not one size?

Sister:
I have come across many brothers who love big women and are not ashamed of their preference. The truth is that by society's "norm," most women (size 12+) are considered full-figured, which any real woman knows is not necessarily true. My advice to you is to get away from brothers that may look to hide their love for you and find a brother who can openly love you. There is no reason that your beauty and passion should not come out to play.

*Y*ep, I am going to jump on the bandwagon and tell you that exercise is good for you. Now, my reasons differ in that I am not at all concerned about the level of your cholesterol, blood pressure, or white-cell count—nope, not interested in those things. I want to make sure that your muscles and other body parts are in prime shape for your ultimate sexual performance. Exercise is key to making sure that you are able to perform at your most stellar level, and it also allows you to literally "bend" with the sexual trends.

So if you have never gotten turned on by the thought of exercise in the past, let me offer up some reasons why it may be the ultimate aphrodisiac:

- You burn up to 300 calories per lovemaking session.

- People who have sex on a regular basis (two to three times per week) often report being happier and more satisfied with the quality of their lives.

- Exercise releases endorphins similar to those given off during an orgasm. Through regular exercise, your body learns to channel these endorphins to extend the level of pleasure.

- Exercise makes your body physically look better, which leads to a sexier perception of self and a desire for more sex.

I think it's time for you to get your exercise thing on in order to have the stamina and stature to attain sexual diva status!

My Personal Path Toward Discovery

Like a lot of sisters out there, I coasted in my early twenties. I could eat anything, and the body was always bikini-ready. For many years I took pride in the fact that while other women woke up at the crack of dawn to hit the gym, I simply rolled over and got another hour of sleep, and when I got to work I looked just as good in a business suit as the workout mavens did in theirs. I didn't exercise because in my mind, I didn't need to.

Since those glory days, I have had two wake-up calls that have changed my attitude when it comes to exercise. A few years ago, when I thought I was "looking my best," I decided to compete in my company's 5k Race for the Cure event. I was just going to walk, so there was no need to train or even exercise beforehand. My co-workers were training every day at lunch, and I was just eating lunch. I thought I could handle this without doing all the prep work others were doing.

Wrong! On the day of the race, I was one of the first to call it quits. I totally misjudged the degree of stamina needed to compete. It wasn't about how thin I looked, but about how healthy I was. I didn't have the athletic ability to keep up.

And then there was the time I started dating "Super Brother." This brother was in the army and in peak physical form. His life was all about how often he could get to the gym and where he was going next to hike, rock climb, or jog. The brother had all of the best jogging and biking paths in the city mapped out, and he was looking for his lady to be able to keep up. Now, honestly, I couldn't have cared less about exercising at this time in my life, but the brother was fine, and I just wanted to get to know him better. So off I went with him to the gym and bike riding, and I think I suffered through one round of racquetball. After three dates, I was pretty good at giving him the impression that I was the dream woman that he had been looking for. The true test came weeks later, when we decided to take our relationship to the next level.

"Super Brother" was simply beautiful; every part of his body was a finely chiseled masterpiece. Sexually, "Super Brother" would last a real long time. When I say a real long time, I mean hours, and with no breaks or downtime. This brother viewed sex as a workout, so it was sex from different angles on the bed, sex on the sex chair, sex on the harness hanging from the ceiling (don't knock it till you try it), and then it went on to sex in the shower. After our first encounter a sister was surprised, but could handle it. Then it got to sex a few times a week, and let's just say a sister was sore and exhausted about halfway through.

LET'S GET IT ON TIP 7

Exercise Your Way to Ecstasy

Use a daily workout plan to boost your sexual stamina, engage sexual muscles, and get into your ultimate sexual form.

How could he keep up this pace? Why wasn't he like other brothers who after about an hour of sex were asleep, or on to something else? This brother had incredible stamina and a huge bag of tricks. His bedroom was a sexual amusement park, and I wasn't tall enough for all of the rides.

But I wanted to be able to keep up with him, so a sister had to get her workout thing on.

As I joined the throngs of people who made the early-morning trek to the gym, I found that my stamina and energy increased. I also began to look more toned and feel more sexy. No longer did "Super Brother" wear me out, and I was able to teach him a few things as well. Unfortunately, when I finally got to the point where I was his sexual match and things were all good, I discovered that he was a little too friendly with his male roommate—*oh well*.

Sexy How-To

My exercise motivation is all about the bedroom—being able to hang in there sexually, look better when naked, and have all of my muscles perfectly toned to do the tricks and flips in bed like booty clapping. And the health benefits are an additional plus!

Here are some fun things to try:

Erotic Exercise

Take a pole or chair class that teaches you the fine art of stripping while giving you better abs and a tighter butt. These classes are fun, because you get so engrossed in learning the technique that you don't realize how much crouching over a chair and giving a lap dance tightens up your thighs. Plus every sister should know how to climb a pole just in case the mood hits her one day.

Belly Dancing

Belly dancing is such a sexy art, and it really teaches you to appreciate the female form in all of its many colors and sizes.

Want great ab control? Belly dancing teaches you the most effective and seductive ways to move your hips and undulate your stomach. You will rotate, girate, and breathe yourself toward the big O.

Pilates/Yoga

Want to step up your sensual side while working out? Take a yoga or Pilates class. Each uses the weight of the body as resistance to tone, shape, and improve flexibility. After an hour of being bent in strange positions and pulled and prodded, you can't help but feel more in touch with your sexual self. The added bonus of these workout routines is flexibility. Remember when you were a teenager and could make love in an economy-sized car or in a twin bed and not live to regret it in the morning? Now is the time to get those days back!

Rock Wall Climbing

I know some of you are going "LaDawn, you have lost your mind! Sisters don't climb walls." Well, you need to look into this one. Climbing has two main benefits: Lots of guys are doing it, and just think of all the great asses you get to see while waiting your turn. You can build your body while checking out others. Plus, wall climbing gives you the stamp of the "adventurous sister," and who couldn't use a little more spice on her résumé?

Spinning

Can you ride a bike? Then spinning may be for you. This is a great exercise to take up if you thrive in a group atmosphere and you were the sister that sucked at aerobics. Spinning is just riding a stationary bike to the rhythm and timing of an instructor. There is so much energy in the class that no one notices if you are just a little off, and because you stay in one place, you can easily enjoy the group dynamic without being thrown off course.

GROUP JOGGING/WALKING TEAMS

This is one of my favorites, because you can exercise while meeting new people with similar interests. Most major cities have jogging/walking/biking teams, and often they are broken down by marital status, ethnic group, or religion, making it easier to join a club that meets your needs. These groups are great because there is a lot of support and they become a community, so there is ample opportunity to get to know people outside of the exercise.

Your Result

Exercise will allow you to be sexier on the outside and sexually competent on the inside. Nature gives us a lot when it comes to sex appeal, but we have to be willing to work hard to maintain what we are given. When you really get out there and get engaged in physical activity, you get to use it for more than just toning and slimming down. Exercise can be used to tighten up your sexual arsenal (stripping), improve the strength of your screw (stronger thighs and better butt), and make doing it all night long a reality (stop thinking it is a myth—some of us actually *can* get it on all night). Learn the secret about exercise that most tight-bodied sisters won't tell you: It is not all about overall health—sometimes it is simply about getting some.

Sexual Toolbox

Kegel exercises are heavily promoted in the media—clenching and releasing the muscles in the vagina that add to the tightness and friction of intercourse. Keep doing your Kegels, but know that there are topical products that can give you instant tightness for twenty-four hours and surgeries that can restore tightness. Visit your local adult novelty store or search online for the latest products and procedures that can bring you back to tighter days.

8

Toy Boys
The New Man Hook

LaDawn:
I can't stop sleeping with other men. My husband has
no idea that I have had a few lovers over the course of
our marriage. Our relationship and sex life are great,
but I just crave the company of new men. Am I a bad
woman for not being faithful, or am I just being real
where other women settle?

Sister:
I am not going to judge whether or not you are good
or bad—that is not my place. Plus, I have been doing
this relationship advice thing long enough to know
that even in the most ideal situations, sometimes you
simply need more. I would encourage you to do some
soul searching, because you really need to understand what these lovers are giving you that your husband isn't. Is the relationship with these lovers not
complicated by bills and children? Are they successful or interesting on a level that your husband isn't, or
do they know you in a way that your husband doesn't
want to or can't see after all the years you've been to-

gether? You have to figure out why you are doing this in order to make a better decision as to whether or not to continue.

*O*kay, I am getting ready to get myself in trouble with this one. I have a personal belief that is going to go against everything that your mom, your church, your girls, and society have told you. I am an advocate for "toy-boy" relationships. Every woman should have at least one relationship in her lifetime that is simply about the sexual hook-up and not about love, commitment, or deeper feelings. Sisters who have had such relationships are saying "amen" right about now, and those that haven't are mortified. I am an advocate for the toy-boy relationship if you are single or in a long-term relationship; there is nothing better to teach you about sex or to revive a sexual fire. Yes, I will admit it, I am officially turning you into a naughty sister.

My Personal Path Toward Discovery

Time to come clean: I have had several toy-boy relationships during my sexual life. There are brothers that you meet where the sexual heat is so apparent that you can care less about where he works, what he thinks about kids, or even that he talks. For me, these relationships seem to come when I am going through a period of major life or career change. There was toy boy 1 when I first moved away from home, toy boy 2 when I got my first apartment, and toy boy 3 when I got out of a disastrous relationship. All of the brothers were fun and brought a different degree of distraction to my life. Sex with these brothers was experimental, invigorating, and fulfilling, because that's all it was. I wasn't looking to fall in love or be with these brothers forever, just to share a moment of their time, and it worked out for all of us in the end.

One particular toy boy was instrumental in teaching me more about sex and sensuality than any long-term boyfriend could. We had been friends for a while, but never could hook up because we were never available at the same time. The next time he came around, I was at a point in a long-term girl-friend/boyfriend situation where I was trying to decide if this was the relationship for me for the long haul. When this particular toy boy came around, it was just like fire—I could not be around him even in public without getting flushed or wanting to touch him. There was no talk about his views on anything or what he thought about me. Personally, I didn't really care—it was all about the sex, and it was grand. This brother introduced me to positions and practices that I'd only read about, and we spent hours at a time in bed. He was all about satisfying me and making a point that I should have been with him years ago. I was all about enjoying the moment and having fun. This hook-up ended like most toy-boy re-

LET'S GET IT ON TIP 8

Get a Toy Boy

Try a sexual relationship with no commitment or future expectations. Live in the moment and rediscover what it's like to just be hot for someone rather than shopping for a soul mate.

lationships do when you realize that the sex isn't enough. So you champion the great experience and get on with the rest of your life.

So how do toy boys benefit you sexually? In my experience, they can put you back in touch with your sexual self. If you have been in a long-term relationship, you often forget what makes you sexy—and toy boys remind you of it daily. They can be great sexual fillers between dates, fulfilling your needs until you get to Mr. Right. Toy boys can give you the ultimate sexual ego boost.

Sexy How-To

So how do you get your very own toy boy? Toy boys come in two forms. There is the brother that you have always been hot for that you knew was never marriage material. It may be time to give this brother a call and find out if he is still interested. Another way to get your very own toy boy is to let the next brother that you hook up with know that you only want him for occasional sex and fun, and that this relationship will be light on feelings and heavy on passion. Trust me—not too many brothers will turn this opportunity down.

Now, the way to make sure that the toy-boy thing works for you is to always keep your feelings out of it—this is a sex thing, and remind him of it constantly. Also, this is the relationship to be experimental in. Do everything with this brother that your man won't do or can't do. This is the fantasy sexual hook-up that will bring about new experiences and new pleasures. And the final key to making the toy-boy thing work is to know when to cut it off. Here are the signs that it is time to end the toy-boy relationship:

- The subject of loving him keeps coming up.
- He wants to know more about your current situation (relationships, career, family, etc.).
- He starts to talk too much about his situation.
- There's too much talk about future activities and plans.
- Either of you wants to talk and bond outside of sex.

These are signs that someone is looking to turn the fun into a full-time relationship. Toy boys are for the moment—a sexual jump-start; rarely are they long-term material.

The final toy-boy tip is for married ladies. I know that the whole toy-boy concept is hard to accept if you are married. How in the world can you cheat on your husband? Personally, I haven't needed a toy boy since I got married, but I have spoken with many a sister that has had these hook-ups and their husbands had absolutely no idea. Why would they jeopardize marriage and family to get a little on the side? There are many reasons:

- To break up sexual monotony
- To explore a sexual side that their husband isn't comfortable with (ménage à trois, anal, role-play, etc.)
- To feel attractive to someone again
- To reclaim a sense of self
- To try out the single life prior to deciding to divorce

In each case, toy boys provide a way of getting your sexual appetite fed and your ego stroked without digging too deep into a relationship. Women who go this route already have a man who is engaged in their lives; what they need is a man who is only concerned with the superficial. Toy boys provide that out.

Your Result

If you choose to add a toy boy to your life, know that the sex will be the hottest that you have had in quite some time. All of the newness and experimentation will reinvigorate your feelings of being sexy and desirable to the opposite sex. You will dress and behave differently as you begin to rediscover your power to sexually please and at times dominate a man. You may also find that your husband or boyfriend becomes more sexually appealing, because subconsciously you want to share with him the tricks and skills that your toy boy has unearthed. These toy-boy relationships are often short, but lead to some of the most memorable times of your sexual life. Get your toy boy today!

Sexual Toolbox

Make a fantasy list. Write out every sexy scenario that you have ever wanted to play out that your last or current man won't, and e-mail it to your toy boy with the message head "Our To-Do List." Make an effort to work through each item on the list, and make sure all of your wildest fantasies are represented.

9

Walk the Red Carpet
Film and Photo

Hey—my man likes to catch me getting out of the shower or getting dressed with his camera phone. I am kind of weirded out by it because the pictures always look bad, and I know that he can easily send the images on his phone to his boys. How can I satisfy his need to record my every naked moment and still protect my right to privacy?

Sister:

Get the brother to stop using the camera phone! Those images are so grainy that I am sure that all of your hotness is not coming through. Invest in a digital camera, so he can snap photos and review them— and you can quickly delete them. I am all for filming your sexcapades, but I always tell sisters to know where the film is. To this day, I hope some of my college exploits don't pop up on the net ☺.

*E*very woman wants to be the center of sexual attention for her man. Many of us have thought about doing a sexy photo spread or filming our next sexual encounter, but decided against it at the last minute because we were too scared of the potential outcome. I am here to tell you, ladies, that recording or photographing sex is an enormous turn-on, because it allows you to see yourself the way a man sees you. You will discover your sexiest parts, best positions, and best angles. You can pose under your man's direction and really get inside his head when it comes to what is really sexy about you.

My Personal Path Toward Discovery

I am a bit of a ham, so this whole thing about photos and videotaping has never been an issue for me. Personally, I always encourage women to go to a professional photographer and have a nude photo taken on milestone birthdays, because it reflects how your confidence and sex appeal change as you age. Nudity should be celebrated, and you should be just as comfortable and confident without a stitch of clothing as you are when you are dressed.

My college boyfriend and I shot a lot of photos and video. He was my man, and because I was young and digital cameras weren't on the scene yet, there is probably a tape somewhere with "LaDawn" on it that someone has long forgotten about. A few years ago he actually sent me the photos to let me know that he wasn't interested in having them anymore, but the tapes weren't returned and at times I am worried, though the truth is they were fun to make and I learned a great lesson back in my freewheeling days from my college boyfriend: that if your man is interested in celebrating and documenting your beauty, you should let him. Some brothers aren't lying to you when they say that you are the most beautiful woman that they have ever seen. If a brother is into

> ## LET'S GET IT ON TIP 9
>
> ### *Learn to Walk the Red Carpet*
>
> Make film your friend.
> Learn to pose and preen
> like a porn star.
> Let your lover capture
> the fantasy for all time.

you, believe me he will treasure these images, and you can celebrate your sexuality through his eyes.

Today I am still into capturing sexual interludes on film. I have posed nude several times both for publication and personal use. I would love to do the video thing, but my man really isn't into that. In our relationship I am the wild one (big surprise there) and he is more careful, so I can be out there naked on film, but you won't catch a glimpse of my man. So while I chase him around the room with my camera phone when he gets out of the shower or spring the digital on him in the middle of the night, I have had to make peace with the fact that I am an exhibitionist married to a more reserved brother. But I am not giving up, because I will get the perfect shot even if we are in our seventies in a nursing home. He will give me my money shot!

Sexy How-To

Because I love being nude, I have discovered different ways to look better when being photographed erotically. The main thing to remember is to relax and enjoy the session and make it fun. If you are being photographed by a pro, make sure that you are comfortable with the person and that you have a clear agreement outlined on how the photos will be used or reprinted. If your man is doing the camera work, come up with ground rules about when you are going to view the images, if and when you will delete them, and whether or not he will share them with his boys. You have to know these things.

Want to look better on film? Here are some surefire tips to put your sexiest diva on shine:

Invest in a gold or silver shimmering lotion.

Give your skin a sparkling boost to add a sexy effect to your image. Shimmer creams make your skin glow, and they can hide cellulite and stretch marks. Also make sure that you apply a coat of baby oil to your skin, which goes a long way toward making you look more toned.

Make sure everything is manicured.

You can't hide a thing when you are naked, so it is important that you are groomed from head to foot. So that means shave, cut down, and polish up every body part. Go for soft hair that can be raked through and easily rearranged even if it is short. Makeup should be soft and sultry. Pay extra attention to the condition of elbows and knees, because many great pictures have gone down the toilet because a sister forgot to smooth these areas out.

Learn to suck it in.

For the hour or so you are taking pictures or being filmed, you have to be conscious of holding in your stomach even if it is flat. Other things to keep in mind: flexing your butt and arms for the ultimate toning effect, and holding your head high in order to avoid any double chin or facial sag. Wear heels no matter what the shot, because they force you to have proper posture and move more seductively.

TRY OUT POSES IN THE MIRROR.

Prior to recording or filming your sexual tryst, practice some poses in the mirror. Have your lover comment on what looks best for those poses that don't allow you to use the mirror. Some ways to manipulate your body for the greatest effect:

Flat belly—lie on your back

Small waist and great ass—lie on your side

Great legs—swing over the side of the bed or wrap them around a chair

Boobtastic—lie flat for a fuller shape that doesn't spill over to the sides

Be creative and make the best use of your sexiest parts.

SET THE MOOD.

Don't forget the atmosphere when it comes to getting your film thing on. You have to create your own set if it is a nude photo or your porn debut. Remember that colored bulbs and candlelight make your skin luminous. Silky fabrics bounce off glimmering skin and can make you feel extra sexy. Pop in your favorite CD to relax you, and make sure your privacy is guaranteed for however long you will need it.

BE THE FANTASY.

Why not try out being a blonde or a redhead for your film debut? Have you ever wanted to play the dominatrix or the servant? Get really crazy with your red-carpet debut by being someone that you are not.

Your Result

I know that taking nude photos and being filmed sexually in the past has allowed me to feel more comfortable in my skin. I know my flaws, but through this sexy exercise I also now know what makes me sexy and different from other sisters. Sisters, hear me closely: Brothers love a great nude image of you. It is a daily reminder of why they got in the relationship in the first place and what they see is theirs to explore. So whether or not you decide to pay a professional to capture your sexiest image or you and your lover break out the old camera late at night, know that this is an opportunity to play the sex-kitten role, and really ham it up for the camera. This is you unhinged, marking a time in your life when you were uninhibited and ready for anything!

SOFT-CORE SEX TIP #3
The Art of Great Conversation

Through your conversation, you can make people feel warm and loved. You can also self-promote and sell yourself in such a way that most people will buy (you) and not even know why. In my opinion, a great conversationalist can win

in any situation because she is able to make people comfortable, keep them entertained, and leave them wanting more.

Sexy How-To

Being a great conversationalist is doing a very delicate dance between learning to both listen and entertain. Also, you have to be diverse in your subject matter in order to have something appropriate to discuss with all people. The final critical point of achieving sexy status when it comes to your conversation is to realize that the best conversationalists know how to draw their audience out whether it is only one person or hundreds—they can make each person feel that their conversation is just for them.

There are three essential ways to jump-start your conversation skills:

- Find common ground
- Soft-promote yourself
- Up-sell

Sexual Toolbox

Start sending erotic photo messages and e-mails to your lover throughout the day. The pictures can be of unexpected G-rated spots on your body: your fingers, your lips, a shoulder, or your hair. Send the image and describe what you plan on doing to him later in the day with that part.

FINDING COMMON GROUND

Finding common ground is easy and pretty clear. If you are doing the one-on-one thing, ask the other person about such broad topics as schools, place of birth, companies worked for, or children. Find something that you have in common, and be creative about how to twist and turn the topic for maximum results. Even when addressing a large crowd, be ready with common experiences that reflect your situation. When I speak to women about relationships, I often open by saying, "I have been through the cycle of bad relationships and I am going to show you how I stopped the cycle." This type of general statement places your audience at ease and lets them know that you have something in common, so you really bond with your audience.

SOFT PROMOTION

You've got to be able to toot your own horn in subtle ways that shine the light on you but do not discount the ideas, accomplishments, or spirit of your audience. There is nothing wrong with talking about your great career, but instead of saying that you are a "super-successful sister," find new ways of conveying your greatness. Mix up your conversation to include the trip that you just took, the landscaping that you had done to your home, or the play that you just saw. Soft promotion works well because it gives people insight into how you live your life without making them feel like underachievers in the process.

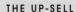

THE UP-SELL

In a conversation it is so important to make others feel that what they are saying and doing is just as important to you as what is going on in your own life. Champion up-sellers know how to get people talking about themselves, and they always have a quick compliment to bestow. They never leave a conversation without building a person or group up, and they never, ever tear themselves down in the process. It is the ultimate way to leave a lasting impression— making others feel good about themselves.

10

Group Love
Ménage à Trois

LaDawn,
I am intrigued with sex clubs and hedonism trips. I think this would be a perfect way to finally get my girl-on-girl fantasy fulfilled. My man is down for the triple play, but I am scared to approach strangers, and the classifieds scare me as well. Do you think these hedonism-type trips are the real deal, or should I just wait until the perfect situation presents itself?

Sister:
The hedonism trips, from what I've heard, are hit-or-miss. Some people live out their greatest fantasies, while others come back saying that it is all a bunch of hype. Like any trip, it may be worth taking if you are referred by someone you trust who had a great time. You may have more luck in the sex clubs. They tend to do what they say they are going to do, the environment is often safe and clean, and privacy is respected. If this is your fantasy, I say definitely go with it.

*L*et's be real: A lot of sisters wonder what it would be like to be with another woman. I can't tell you how many women share this fantasy with me at night on the radio. Most ladies get turned on by the image of two women making love but are quick to say that it isn't really anything that they want to do. Other women have been incredibly honest about how they have relationships with women that sometimes involve their men, and how these sexual encounters have taught them to appreciate the female form and learn better ways to be pleased.

There are also sisters out there who want a ménage à trois with more than one man—no extra girl needed. I had a sister write to me about her wild nights with her man and his best friend and how she had never been turned out or on like that. I stand by the sister who is able to pull the two-man thing off. Where are the brothers who are open to this? I teased my man one night with this scenario and he looked at me as if my head had just split open and aliens had popped out. So let's just say I am always impressed when a sister is able to pull off this minor miracle.

If you have ever wondered what it would be like to throw a third into the mix, then stop wondering about it and get into the mix. A ménage à trois can introduce you to sexual play and broaden your pleasure horizons.

My Personal Path Toward Discovery

I think that women are beautiful, and I can appreciate a great body as much as any guy. Now, before you start thinking that this is a coming-out tale, know that if most women were honest, they would admit to having the same fascination with the female form. We are almost brainwashed to be attracted to female beauty by all the magazines, movies, and books that focus on the female form. That is why I think that bringing another woman as a third into the bedroom is not a bad thing. I haven't done it yet, but I wouldn't run from the prospect if it presented itself. In my mind, it is an experience to have and not a declaration of my sexual preference.

In the case of having two men, this idea has intrigued me for some time, and as I said, I actually presented it to my man. It didn't fly, but I haven't given up. Who knows what can happen down the road?

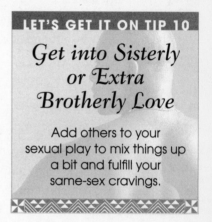

LET'S GET IT ON TIP 10

Get into Sisterly or Extra Brotherly Love

Add others to your sexual play to mix things up a bit and fulfill your same-sex cravings.

Sexy How-To

So how do you get your ménage on? Let me walk you through three key steps in the process:

IS IT WHAT YOU WANT?

The first step toward getting your group thing on is to evaluate if this is really what you want. Are you doing this to please your partner, or because you crave it? Are you comfortable sharing your lover? What if word of the tryst gets out? Could you handle that? All of these are important questions to answer prior to entering the bedroom. You want to be relaxed and ready for pleasure and not nervous and edgy when the day arrives.

SET THE GROUND RULES.
Once you have decided to move forward, it is time to establish rules for the threesome. Discuss whether or not your man gets to watch or participate. Is this a one-time-only arrangement, or will threesomes be a regular occurrence in your relationship? Will the third party be a friend or a stranger? Talk this out prior to the sexual act.

FIND A THIRD.
Where can you find a third party? If you want to be selective, you can use a classified ad or hire a pro. You can easily specify what type of person you are looking for and clearly define the rules of your sex play. If you want your encounter to be a little more casual, try a sex club to meet that third. At these clubs you often meet and mingle on one level, like at any regular networking event, and then move on to another level in the house or club and get to know one another more intimately. Also, use the Internet to search out swinging clubs, message boards, and hook-up sites.

Your Result

Adding a third (or fourth) to your love life will give you the opportunity to step into the world of fantasy. You will experience something that most people only talk about. The added bonus is that you get to share this unique sexual experience with someone you love and trust, on your terms.

Sexual Toolbox

Want to freak a man out? Instead of opting for just another sister in the room, why not surprise him with twins? Pick a sister who is similar to you in looks, and double his pleasure and his fantasy with a threesome where he sees double.

11

The Diva's Den

Getting It On in Your Boudoir

LaDawn:
I only like making love at my place and not at my man's. Is this strange? I get creeped out by how many women he may have had in his bed, and also he isn't quite as clean as I would like him to be. How can I get past this?

Sister:
Why are you stressing over how many sisters this brother has had in his bed? You knew he wasn't a virgin when you first sexed him, so you are going to have to grow up a little and accept that there have been other women not only in his sheets but all over his body as well. As far as locking yourself down in your place, you are limiting your relationship. A person's home says so much about him or her, and the fact that he wants you in his space is his way of letting you know that he trusts you and has nothing to hide. So get down off your super-clean high horse and make the trek over to his place for occasional nookie. If you

plan on being with this brother for the long haul, you have to make peace with his way of living right now.

*L*adies, I am going to give you the inside scoop on a male pet peeve that you may not be aware of: Most of them hate your bedroom. They don't find your space sexy or comfortable. Often they feel out of place and unwanted. I hear from so many brothers that women have lost the art of seduction, and setting the stage for sex in the bedroom is usually the top gripe. Actually, I have a good friend who won't sex a woman if there are any stuffed animals or live pets in the room. Crazy-sounding, I know, but the brother sees the stuffed animals as representing a little girl not wanting to grow up and a pet as something else competing for a woman's attention when he should be the most important thing at the moment. It's time to get your bedroom in top shape for love.

My Personal Path Toward Discovery

I remember when I learned how important it was to set the stage for sex. I had just moved into my first place, and I thought I had decorated my house with top skill. Everything was new, and I was excited to show off my handiwork. The first time I invited a brother over I gave him the grand tour, and when we got to the bedroom he laughed. When I asked what was so funny, he quickly stated that no man was ever going to sleep in this bedroom because he couldn't get around all the stuffed animals. I had a whole wall dedicated to every stuffed animal I had collected since birth. On top of that I had a lot of sentimental keepsakes and cards to remind me of special times in my life. The brother said that I had a shrine to LaDawn in my bedroom. In his mind, this room would never be sexy.

After several starts and stops with bedroom decorating, I have finally found my idea of a seductive bedroom that won't send the brothers running for the nearest exit. My particular formula is a mix of gender-neutral design elements, erotic accents, and making sure there is nothing in there to interfere with the mood. Even though I'm married, I still keep the bedroom ultra-sexy. Although we women often call the shots when decorating, it is still important to remember that a man will inhabit the space.

Sexy How-To

Don't let a simple thing like bedroom design kill your sexual mood. Here are six tips for creating an ultra-sexy boudoir that will entice him to keep coming back:

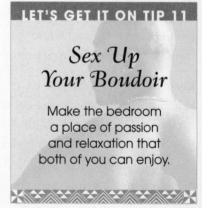

LET'S GET IT ON TIP 11

Sex Up Your Boudoir

Make the bedroom a place of passion and relaxation that both of you can enjoy.

PLAY ON THE BIG SWING.
Invest in an adult bed that is formidable and stylish—no canopies or futons. So many men complain that women tend to go for pretty little beds that don't look strong or inviting.

Think dark wood, fabric headboards, and a bed that sits high off the floor. A grown-up bed for grown-folk activities.

INVEST IN A GOOD CHEST.

Anything that is furry, makes a noise, or has plastic eyes should go into a keepsake chest. Also stash anything that an old boyfriend may have given you. Memories are great, but your new lover wants a clean slate and not to feel that he is corrupting your Barbie collection.

REMOVE THE DISTRACTIONS.

Take the television and the office out of the bedroom. Make your bedroom a place of relaxation or sexual play. If you allow a television in, the room turns into a den and not a sexual oasis. If your office is in the bedroom, you may just decide to hop on the computer instead of rolling over for fifteen more minutes of cuddling. Define your space by removing any elements that detract from passion.

KISS THE FLOWERS AND ANIMAL PRINTS GOOD-BYE.

When it comes to actually decorating your room, stay away from pastel walls and any kind of lace; these are girly elements that are sure to make him feel less than manly. Also, when choosing patterns, stay away from animal prints, which most men find unflattering, and any sort of flower that screams "woman living alone!" Try paisley, stripes, and unique solid colors. Make the room décor an environment that says "I want to share my space with you" and not "Hello Kitty."

MAKE A LOVE OASIS.

Add simple touches to set the mood like candles, fresh flowers, and beautiful makeup and brush trays that show your unique style. Have all of your favorite scents and lotions displayed and close by for a great massage or quick misting. If you are like me and you constantly have robes lying out, make sure they are lush and sexy. These small touches really add up.

Keep toys around.

Every room should have a playful aspect. I suggest that every sister have a toy drawer or box in the bedroom filled with love goodies. This should be your go-to drawer for protection, massage oils, lubricants, feathers, and vibes. Maybe even add a sexy CD or a small camera to your collection. Instead of having to look for a playful item when you are in the mood, have them close at hand.

Your Result

This tip is common sense. If you want to have a better sex life, make sure that your room's décor supports it. Now, I know that if you want to get your freak on, you can do it anywhere—under any circumstances. However, what separates the average sister from the hottest sister is the presentation and prep work. It's not all about the makeup and hair, it is also about the beauty and texture of your space and how welcoming it is to a man looking to be with you. Just think about that great guy you once met only to realize when you went back to his place that he had not thrown away a *Jet* magazine since 1984. Remember how fast you came up with ways to get out of his space? What makes you think he doesn't look at your Care Bear and feel the same way?

Sexual Toolbox

In your sexual toy drawer, make sure there is at least one toy for him. Throw a vibrating cock ring in the mix and learn how to work it properly. Always present it as something you got just for him (even if it has seen quite a few users).

Necessary Pain

Bite and Claw Your Way to Passion

LaDawn:
My man bit the hell out of my nipple the other day and I thought that my screams would tell him that this wasn't really the way to turn me on. Last night he tried it again and he just kept biting me and getting more and more turned on by my obvious displeasure. Are brothers into the whole S&M thing? I thought this was the kink of strange white people!

Sister:
Your man is definitely turned on by handing out pain. You need to talk to him about what he wants to do, and be clear and honest with him about what you are willing to do. It is important that you come to an agreement that works for both of you. I caution you, though, not to make the brother feel as if his turn-on is strange or not "brother-like." We all are turned on by things that others may view as strange, but the world is big enough for consenting adults to get their freak on in as many ways as we can come up with. For every fetish or freakish fascination that you think is

"white," simply do an Internet search and you will find an African-American site dedicated to the same practice. We are quite a freaky bunch!

*K*inky sex is often the best sex! Forget missionary and doggy-style and familiarize yourself with the world of the dominatrix (sexual domination), golden shower aficionado (turned on by urination), and walking the dog (sex in the park with strangers). If this is all a little too wild for you, then maybe we should start you out with simply being more aggressive in bed. There is so much more than a kiss and penetration when it comes to sex. With a simple bite, twist, or lick, you can make the average encounter an extraordinary one.

My Personal Path Toward Discovery

Every sister should be lucky enough to get a "trick boy"—a brother who is always looking to be different in bed. A trick boy is the one who always wants it in public places, in strange positions, and with unique flavors attached. Often this is the brother who introduces you to the world of kink. This is the brother who researches and refines his sex and can't wait to try his new discovery out on you.

My trick boy was fascinated with causing pain. Now, he wasn't hard-core with whips, chains, or nails—he specialized in light pain for ultimate pleasure. Before we slept together for the first time, he shared with me this particular turn-on and a sister wasn't really interested in moving forward. I have a very low tolerance for pain, and at the time I believed a little bit of hurt would eventually turn into a huge amount. It took quite a bit of convincing for me to let him do everything that he wanted to do to me. This brother's main

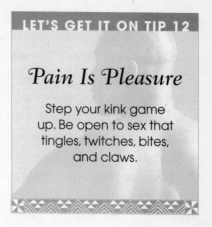

LET'S GET IT ON TIP 12

Pain Is Pleasure

Step your kink game up. Be open to sex that tingles, twitches, bites, and claws.

attraction was to bite parts of my body gently. When he first came at me with his teeth, I just knew that I was going to be in the emergency room trying to explain to the doctor why I willingly let a man turn me into an entrée.

But once I relaxed and surrendered to his fantasy, I realized this brother wasn't an amateur biter, he was skilled. His bite was gentle and electric. He knew exactly how much pressure to use and where to place it. I was then open to his other sexy suggestions. This brother did not only bring the pain; he was also masterful with feathers. He was all about the sensations of the skin and bringing different ways of touch to the table. Trust me, you haven't lived until you have given yourself over to a brother who is telling you what he wants to do to you while tracing your body with a feather. Corny? Maybe. Hot? Definitely!

Sexy How-To

Before Trick Brother, I wasn't really up on all of the many fetishes and tricks out there to enhance your sexual experiences. Luckily, I met him early on and I was able to stay literally on top of new games, positions, and sexual trends to maximize sexual stimulation. The easiest way to find out what type of kinky activity fits your needs is to do some research. The first step is to really get down to what turns you on that you haven't shared with anyone. One sister that called my radio show admitted that she enjoyed meeting random men and having sex—no names, conversation, or future expectations. Her husband wasn't into this, so she had to find ways to feed her desire on her own. After a quick ad search in her town's party paper, she found a weekly sex party that guaranteed anonymity and the opportunity to meet and hook up several times a night. Her kink hunger was satisfied. Here are some steps to get you in touch with your kinkier side:

What are your triggers?

What turns you on? Always be on the lookout for films and articles that entice you. Information is king, and being able to tie in the fact that you enjoy prolonged foreplay with a desire to learn more about Tantric sex is crucial to making sure that you are fulfilling your every desire.

What do you hide from others sexually?

Another way of identifying what you want to explore sexually is to really think hard about the sexual self that you hide from your lover or friends. Is there something that turns you on or an experience that you want to relive that you keep private? The secret turn-on of one sister I know is watching men masturbate. She discovered this with a boyfriend who could only climax by jerking off. At first she wondered if she wasn't enough woman for him, but then she realized that this was his sexual turn-on and it soon became hers as well. Years later, while watching porn with other men, she found herself still turned on by the voyeuristic aspects of watching a man please himself. When she finally made peace with her kink, she was able to share it with future lovers who were more than willing to supply her with the images she needed to get off.

After identifying your kink, you need to find out where to go to feed your appetite.

Start at home.

Let your lover or any potential lovers know what really turns you on. Invite them into your fetish world and expand your sexual menu. You never know—your partner may have the same appetite or have ideas on how to get you fed.

Search the Internet.

Looking for others turned on by dry humping (believe me, I had a whole radio show on this one), all you have to do is a simple Internet search and a world of dry humpers will open up for you. You can search for dry humpers in your town, break them down by race, or even look for first-timers instead of pros. The Internet literally puts every fetish at your fingertips.

Use message boards.

Once you find the Internet site, make sure you get active in the chat room or message board. Use these as tools to gather more information on what turns you on, meet people interested in sharing your experience, and get great info on conferences and clubs that facilitate your fantasy.

CHECK OUT FREE CITY WEEKLIES.

Most cities have a free weekly that is full of club and activity info. Usually way in the back, buried with your typical man-seeking-woman and woman-seeking-man ads, are the fun ones where individuals are looking for others of like mind to get their freak on with. Also, you can often find local classes to train you in new sexual techniques and the art of seduction.

Your Result

We all have a kinky side. Personally, I am a bit of an exhibitionist and love sex in public places, so I make sure that I get a little taste of my kink in order to stay fulfilled. Don't be shy about your turn-ons, and make sure any lover knows how to please you in the way that you desire. One of the keys to being satisfied is to become familiar with groups, associations, and information sites that provide outlets for your sexual expression. Remember, all is fair when consenting adults decide to engage in sexual play.

Sexual Toolbox

Into spanking? Why not vary your implements of painful pleasure? You can always use your hand, but also consider belts, whips, paddles, and even spoons. Each tool leaves a different type of mark and provides varying levels of sensation.

SOFT-CORE SEX TIP #4

Sample Life's Many Pleasures

When was the last time you took off for the weekend, tried a new restaurant, or tried out a new hobby or interest? Have you reached outside your circle to forge a new friendship or to experience a new culture? Have you taken the time to actually sit and take in your surroundings and bask in their beauty and clarity? We are talking here about really breathing in life and developing great stories and vantage points that will fuel your very special appeal.

Sexy How-To

How exactly do you start living your fuller life? You have to start with simply developing a spirit of wanting to do so. The next time you read a great article about a great locale or hobby, why not look into getting signed up? Another thing to try is to write down a list of items that you would like to try. Slowly work your way down the list until all of the items are checked off. Develop a spirit that screams yes instead of one that is constantly searching for a reason to say no.

Finally, surround yourself with people who also want to try new things, and watch your energy and interests grow. You will be amazed how much your energy level can shift just because you are around the right people.

13

Around the World

Erogenous Zone Tour

YOUR QUESTION

LaDawn:
I listened to the show last night and I could not believe
that people were talking about armpit fucking. Are
you serious? I wish some dude would try to stick his
dick under my arm. It would be on.

Sister:
As strange as underarms may sound, I have heard of
even more incredible friction points on the body.
Brothers have called in with their stories of ear, nose,
and chin sex. All of these things seem pretty strange,
but apparently they're possible.

We focus so much on the penis, breasts, anus,
vagina, and mouth as erotic zones that we forget that skin covers our entire bodies and is
sensitive all over. There are so many parts on the body that can

be licked and caressed to bring pleasure. Sexed-up individuals know that a hand on a shoulder or a lick between the shoulder blades can be just as erotic as a kiss on the lips. It is all about location, pressure, and intent. You can rub, suck, and tease every inch of the body and drive your lover wild.

My Personal Path Toward Discovery

I remember being in high school and really taking the time to make out with my boyfriend. I mean, we tried to do everything that we could do outside of actually having intercourse. This was a time of great learning for me because it was my first real sexual introduction, and because I wasn't going all the way, it forced me to learn different ways to please him outside of traditional intercourse.

As I matured sexually, it became clear that foreplay was not just a precursor to intercourse—it was a way to really get to know your lover's body before being one with it. I learned this lesson from a particular brother who took his sexuality in steps and wanted to see and touch everything. There was no rush to his game, and he took extreme pleasure in learning my body and encouraging me to explore his. This brother went on a world tour of my body and through him, I discovered that the underside of my breasts was sensitive and the small of my back was incredibly ticklish, and I loved for him to lick me there. I discovered his sexy inner thighs and that this brother was incredibly turned on by having his fingers and toes kissed and sucked (don't act like you've never thought to do this).

When we got together, nothing was rushed and there was

always time to discover something new sexually. The time he went from going down on me to actually licking my anus, I thought I was going to literally fly off the bed. It was an area that I had never thought to explore, but when he went there it was well worth it. To this day he is "butt boy"—not the most flattering nickname, I know, so let's keep it between us.

Sexy How-To

There are many ways to do this exploration. The important thing is to do it with every lover and keep it going throughout your relationship. Here are some fun ways to get your exploration started:

EDIBLE BODY PAINTS

I can't think of a better way to explore a person's body than to integrate sexy artwork, touch, and tasty treats—all things that I love. Go to your favorite adult site or store and purchase edible paint or chocolate cream, and get to stroking your lover's body with it. You may discover that his ankles are particularly sensitive, or perhaps his shoulders. Lie back and allow him to return the favor, and close your eyes and simply follow the sensations.

> **LET'S GET IT ON TIP 13**
>
> ## Discover New Erogenous Zones
>
> Take the time with every lover to explore each other's body with the lights on and no expectations of completing the act. Discover curves, creases, and sensations that have been ignored or dormant for some time.

CANDLE WAX

Invest in plenty of slow-burning candles and drip your lover toward ecstasy. For an added heightener, alternate between the heat of the wax and the chill of an ice cube. Maybe throw some handcuffs or a scarf into the mix as a restraint. There are some great candles on the market that actually melt down into a great massage cream for further sexual investigation. It is all about discovering new sexual horizons.

MASSAGE

Forget your typical massage that kneads the muscles. Why not brush up on more seductive techniques? Use your nails as a massage implement, softly tracing your lover's body all over with a tingly touch. Or try my favorite massage technique: Use your body as the massager. Slowly run your nipples, hair, and vagina all over his body while not letting him touch you. See how he reacts to the friction of your body and double your pleasure through feeling his body against your skin. Most men want all massages to turn naughty—give him the fantasy.

FEATHERS AND SILK

Add silky scarves and feathers to your next foreplay session. It is great to run them over the skin, but don't forget to also glide them between the legs, over the nipples, and along closed eyes and lips. Get the whole lover in the game.

GETTING YOUR HANDS DIRTY

For some, the old way of exploring the body is best, and that is with the fingers and tongue. To update this traditional pleasure-seeking mission, be sure to add honey dust, warming creams, or flavored lubricant.

Your Result

There are so many areas on the body that are sensitive to touch, taste, and smell that you can't just stop at the money parts. Also, it is important to note that each of us is different, and what turns one person on may not do it for another. Each new lover presents you with a full-blown quest to discover new pleasure points. Even in long-term relationships, you have to take the time to reacquaint yourself with your lover's hot spots. All of this research has everything to do with turning a lover out in ways that he has never been turned out before. And we all know a good turning-out is priceless as far as keeping a person coming back for more.

Sexual Toolbox

Instead of exploring your lover's body while lying down, why not try it standing up in front of a full-length mirror? This way you are able to see his expression as you discover new pressure points, and he can have the added sexiness of watching you please him.

14
Wanna Get High
Buzzed Sex

Note: *I am not supporting the use of drugs and alcohol as sexual aids. This chapter simply speaks to a common sexual state.*

YOUR QUESTION

LaDawn:
Girl, the other night I think I had a wet dream. I had the most vivid images of making love to my man when he wasn't even at my place that night. I had an orgasm in my sleep, and when I woke up I was really feeling the after-effects. Can women have wet dreams? I always thought our plumbing was different from men's and this was impossible. I think that will be the last time I take a sleeping pill after a night on the town.

Sister:
Please know that you are indeed able to have a purely mental orgasm based on imagery, just like a man. This is especially possible if you are a very visual lover who is turned on by seeing and taking in the sexual experience rather than being a silent participant. I encour-

age you to dig deeper into your pleasure potential through self-pleasure. There really are no limits to what you can accomplish alone.

I have had drunk sex! Some of my best experiences have been when both of us were just a little inebriated and in the most silly and strangely passionate ways ripping each other's clothes off. Look, when a brother is normally a little reserved sexually and you hunger for a wild lover, there is nothing like a little drink or smoke to lure him over to the dark side.

My Personal Path Toward Discovery

I am going to be totally honest here: There have been times when a little liquid courage went a long way toward turning a friend into a lover, letting me approach the hot brother in the club, or simply getting my freak on in a new and exciting way. Most women won't admit to using a bit of an extra push because of its slutty or freak connotation, but since I talk sex with strangers five nights a week, I gave up a long time ago on the whole good-girl thing.

The truth about buzzed sex is that whether your high of choice is in liquid, pill, or leaf form, it allows you to put to rest inhibitions and really get on with experiencing life. Now, before the pure-hearted jump on me, saying that I am advocating addiction, know that I am not talking about hard-core users, just those of us who like to have a "good time" on occasion.

Sexy How-To

Typically, I would walk you through the "how to" of a particular sexual tip, but I am confident that you already know what gets you high and how to use it. Instead I am going to give you some interesting things to try the next time you are slightly buzzed and getting ready to have sex. Now that I think about it, this may be a total waste of ink because if you are high you won't remember it, but on the off chance you turn into a sexual savant when high, here are some things you may want to try:

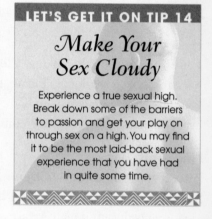

LET'S GET IT ON TIP 14

Make Your Sex Cloudy

Experience a true sexual high. Break down some of the barriers to passion and get your play on through sex on a high. You may find it to be the most laid-back sexual experience that you have had in quite some time.

GET YOUR STRIP ON.

Use your high to give a private peep show. Take the opportunity to dance for your lover or allow him to pose you and direct you sexually while you are on the bed and he watches from a chair in the room.

HAVE BACKYARD SEX.

Take your sex outside to the backyard and get your freak on. Make your movie fantasy come true—roll around in the grass or make love under the stars. Don't limit yourself to the back-yard. Think about all the public places where you yearn to make love and do it!

EXPLORE FANTASY ISLAND.

What has been your most forbidden fantasy? Now may be the time to unleash it and make it a reality. Use your open-minded state to take those naughty photos, have sex with that dumb but hot guy, or hook up with your ex. Enjoy the session and then write it off the next day as "one of those nights."

HAVE SENSORY SEX.

Let your senses do the talking. Close your eyes, lie back, and have the sex be the focus. Luxuriate in the feelings of having your lover tour and tease your body. A subtle buzzing can make every tickle and tingle feel incredible.

HAVE AN AFFAIR.

After a night out, instead of just going back home or to his place, why not check into a cheap hotel just for the purpose of having a tawdry affair night? Have an affair with your lover and snatch the soap and towels in the morning.

Your Result

Buzzed sex will allow you to do it all and blame it on the high the next day. Live out your fantasies, hook up with your fantasy lover, and make the sensations of sex take center stage. Having sex on a high should not be your go-to move, but it can indeed be a sporadic treat to give your life a boost in the hotness di-rection.

Sexual Toolbox

The next time you have your buzz on, up the euphoria with a colored lightbulb or background music in a foreign language. Invest in a light that mimics a starry night sky. You can really have sex that is out of this world.

15

Fire Starter

Long-Term Relationships

LaDawn:

I have been married for eleven years and I don't care what anyone says—sex isn't as hot today as it was when we were dating and first married. I have two kids and two jobs, and don't have the time to really invest in sex. I am tired, and I get tired of people calling your show saying that women don't want sex—I want it, I just don't have time for it. What can you do to keep the fire burning when you are just trying to make it through your day?

Sister:

The first step to heating up your sex life is to stop making excuses! When you first met your man you had a life, but you found a way to make him feel special and I am quite sure he did the same for you. It is all about wanting to do it and deciding to get it done. One night a month, give the kids to someone else and cook a dinner for just the two of you, play your favorite music or watch a movie, dance together and simply reconnect. Place a limit on career and kid talk and focus on what you desire for the future and what you want from each other. Make the night about the two of you and make it count.

I am an advocate of feeding your long-term relationship because if Mom and Dad aren't happy, neither is the rest of the family. Sex is an important part of a relationship and you have to put forth the effort to make it happen on the regular. It may seem like work at first, but it will soon turn into a great way to begin and/or end the day.

*Y*ou would be surprised at the number of people who e-mail and call me regarding loveless and sexless long-term relationships. According to my radio listeners and readers, there are a lot of folks out there not getting any, or feeling that their relationships aren't worth saving. I have always wondered what happens between the time when a couple can't keep their hands off of each other and the point when absolutely nothing loving is going on in their house. What is the secret of the long-term couple that manages to stay connected and fulfilled? Did they simply pick a better mate, or is it more than just natural attraction?

My Personal Path Toward Discovery

I am confessing that after more than ten years of being with the same person, there have been times in our relationship when not all of the burners have been hot. Once, right after our son was born, we considered it a sexy night if we both managed to take a shower and watch *CSI*. Another time we were on a sexual downturn was when we were both working so hard that we simply were never in the same place.

I learned a long time ago from a good married older friend that "a couple that ain't sexing ain't gonna last." Kind of a crass way to look at a loving relationship, but I got what she was saying. A long-term relationship takes the same degree of planning and nurturing that a dating relationship often gets automatically. In my case, I had to learn the value of keeping it sexy all the time. That meant throwing away the comfort drawers, ugly bras, and baggy painter's jeans. It also meant working on the emotional and mental aspects of my relationship. I had to let my man know daily that I loved him, why I loved him, and what I thought was sexy and interesting about him. When I put in this degree of work he began to feed it back to me, and we soon realized that married sex can indeed be hot—it just takes some effort and getting out of the comfortable mode.

A friend of mine actually moved out of her house because she was tired of being taken advantage of and ignored by her man. She left the kids there with him. After about a week, he realized how much she contributed to his home life and started to pay her more attention and devote more time to the relationship. For six months, she lived the life of a single woman who was heavily courted by her

> **LET'S GET IT ON TIP 15**
>
> ## Feed the Fire of Long-Term Love
>
> Keep your sex muscle healthy by constantly trying to up the sexual ante with dates, games, and seduction scenarios. Don't take your sex life for granted.

husband. She eventually moved back into the house, and there was a new dedication on both their parts to keeping the relationship sexy and a top priority.

Sexy How-To

Every relationship needs a sexual jump-start from time to time. Here are five ways to get the charge that you need:

MAKE IT A NIGHT.

As trite as it may seem, it is great to plan date nights a few times during the month when the evening is all about the two of you doing something that you love to do. Ban talk about jobs, bills, and kids and really focus on the friendship between you. Rediscover why you have been with your lover for so long and discover new and surprising facts and stories about him.

FOCUS ON THE POSITIVE.

On a daily basis, reacquaint yourself with what your lover has over any other person. Identify all of his great traits and make sure that you let him know what you find exciting, sexy, and interesting about him. Often as a relationship matures, we forget the power of flattering words and just assume that our partner knows how we feel. Voicing our feelings reinforces our belief in them and lets our partner know that there is still value in the relationship.

SEDUCE AT WORK.

Remember the days when there were sexy calls, e-mails, and text messages throughout the day? Do you even do this anymore? Is there anticipation about the evening ahead? Do you ever call to just thank your lover for the morning session of sex? It is so sexy to be in a totally unsexy situation and be reminded of how desirable you are by a person who actually matters. Make the hours that you are away from each other really count by seducing each other throughout the day.

REFRESH YOUR LOOK.

One of the best ways to jump-start a sexual rebirth is to change your look. When you look sexy, you are more likely to pursue sexy activities. We all get into a rut, and the best way to bust up an old attitude is to gain a new one through a change in hair, makeup, and clothes. Why not get a couple do-over where you and your lover individually choose new looks and present them for one night only? This can add a whole new dimension to your relationship, in which you get insight into how your lover sees you and what he wishes to see down the road.

WALK DOWN MEMORY LANE.

Pull out the videos, pictures, and keepsakes from days past and walk down memory lane. Reacquaint yourself with your shared history and all of the love and excitement in the past. This is the ultimate refresher course on why you love each other today and what you hope for the future.

Your Result

It is so easy these days to move out of a relationship that isn't fulfilling or giving us the juicy feelings that it may have in the past. At times it's not even because you aren't having sex anymore, it is because you know what to expect from the session and there is no warm-up or foreplay involved; you just want to get the sex in before you get on to the rest of your day. There was a time when you spent all day in bed and there was no one that you wanted to see more at the end of the day because you could smell, taste, and feel his lips on you all day long. You can recapture those feelings of passion, but it takes work and dedication to getting your sex game up. Relationships aren't on autopilot, and neither is your sex life. Plan the seduction and the follow-through and you can't help but see a spark return.

Sexual Toolbox

Draw up a twelve-month plan to shock your lover. Mix in new sex toys, fantasy fulfillment, wigs, positions, and much more. It's time to seduce your lover.

SOFT-CORE SEX TIP #5
Celebrate Hotness in Others

Do you want to make others feel great about you? This is an old idea that still holds true today: Get people talking about themselves. If you can make people feel great about themselves, they will never leave your side. You turn into a superhero who is such a great girl.

There is a definite trick to this that I am going to teach you. Once you get a person to open up using this trick, you will never, ever be able to lose. Bringing forth your very own sexiness often involves also shining a light on others.

Sexy How-To

It is so easy to make others feel like sexual superstars. Whenever you are out socially, don't hesitate to acknowledge what you like about them or find appealing. It can be as simple as a piece of jewelry, clothes, hair, or a great car. You can dig deeper and simply love a person's passion for causes, attention to detail, or sexy voice. Every person has an element that is appealing, and true sexual divas know how to shine the light on the positive.

Now, this tip does not apply only to sisters trying to gain the attention of, or leave an impression on, a great brother. To really win the sexy race, you have to use this on women as well. This is actually my specialty. By complimenting other women on their appearance, you are letting them know that you appreciate their unique beauty and that you are not intimidated by it. In many ways you elevate your own sex appeal, because your game is so tight that you have no issues with identifying and praising another sister. If you can make sisters in a social situation comfortable with you, then you are free to work your sexual magic on any eligible brother in the room because you then turn into the sexy sister who "doesn't know how sexy she really is."

Sexy Enough for You?
Wrapping It All Up

LaDawn:
I think about doing it all the time. Am I an addict, or just oversexed? I don't cheat, but honestly at times I can't get enough. My girlfriends are laid back when it comes to sex, but I can't wait to get my next dose.

Sister:
Embrace your sexual self. There is nothing wrong with wanting sex often and in every possible way. The key is to work your fantasy world into your reality. Make sure your lover is able to keep up with you and don't shut him out. Believe me—the brother will be crazy about your robust appetite!

*D*o you have your whips and fantasies ready? Are you getting your Tae Bo on and letting out your inner kink? Have you thought about the guy in the mailroom and whether or not he is your very own "toy boy"? If so, you are so getting it on! The overall message in this book is that life is too short to not be getting the quality and quantity of sex that you deserve. By simply changing your attitude toward sex and marrying that attitude to some new tricks, you can greatly improve the passion in your life.

Each woman has the power within to get exactly what she wants from any lover and give it back a hundred times over. You just have to be honest about what you want, research and try new things, and make a commitment to never give up on your sexual self. A great sex life is so much more than just the ultimate orgasm; it is about physical and mental well-being, connecting with others, understanding the world you live in, and occasionally turning someone out. What fun!

As with all of my books, *Let's Get It On* has a lot to do with my own journey toward my ultimate sexual self. While I have mastered quite a few of the tips here, there are others that I am growing into, but I will never stop my sexual study—it's not fair to me or my lover. So I encourage you to take the tips and use them as you deem appropriate for your level of freakiness, and I guarantee that you will have some of the hottest sex ever.

Let's get it on!

—L

Let's Get It On
Sex Tip Cheat Sheet

BE THE SEXUAL ANNIHILATOR

Give yourself a sexual jump-start. Learn something new and implement it.

START TO REALLY LIKE MEN

Work on getting to know and really appreciate brothers.

PERSONAL CARE

Sweat the small stuff. Stay smooth, fragrant, and soft.

ASK HIM WHAT HE WANTS

Don't assume all men want the same things.

GET IN THE GAME

Add a sense of play to your sexual activity.

PERFECT YOUR ORAL FORM

A blow job is more than just lips and a tongue.

EXERCISE YOUR WAY TO ECSTASY

Use a daily workout plan to boost your sexual stamina, engage sexual muscles, and get into your ultimate sexual form.

GET A TOY BOY
Try a sexual relationship with no commitment or future expectations.

LEARN TO WALK THE RED CARPET
Make film your friend. Learn to pose and preen like a porn star.

GET INTO SISTERLY OR EXTRA BROTHERLY LOVE
Add others to your sexual play to mix things up a bit and fulfill your same-sex cravings.

SEX UP YOUR BOUDOIR
Make the bedroom a place of passion and relaxation that both of you can enjoy.

PAIN IS PLEASURE
Be open to sex that tingles, twitches, bites, and claws.

DISCOVER NEW EROGENOUS ZONES
Take the time with every lover to explore each other's body with the lights on and no expectations of completing the act. Discover curves, creases, and sensations that have been ignored or dormant for some time.

MAKE YOUR SEX CLOUDY
Break down some of the barriers to passion and get your play on through sex on a high.

FEED THE FIRE OF LONG-TERM LOVE
Keep your sex muscle healthy by constantly trying to up the sexual ante with dates, games, and seduction scenarios.

Want more information on relationships?

Log on to www.ladawnblack.com for:
- Love Q & A
- Tour Info
- Message Boards
- Video Relationship Advice
- Dating Events
- And much more . . .

Make www.ladawnblack.com your relationship portal!

About the Author

A native of Washington, D.C., LaDawn Black is a relationship expert, author, and TV/radio personality. Black is the host and producer of Baltimore's number-one radio relationship show, "The Love Zone," on 92Q(92.3FM). She is also the host of one of Baltimore's hottest lifestyle/entertainment television shows, *Keepin' It Real.* In 2005 she was named Baltimore's Best Radio Personality by the *Baltimore City Paper.* Black also contributes relationship advice to blackmeninamerica.com and match.com, and has been featured in *Ebony, Essence, Jewel Magazine,* and *Baltimore Magazine. Let's Get It On* is her second relationship guide. Black resides in Baltimore, Maryland, with her two very best black men, JB and Alec. Visit her website at www.ladawnblack.com.